Livonia Public Library
Livonia Civic Center Library
32777 Five Mile Rd.
Livonia, MI 48154-3045
(734) 466-2491
LIVN #19

PROSTATE
CANCER

FROM THE SAME PUBLISHER
(apediteur.com)

In the same collection

Fred Saad, MD, and Michael McCormack, MD
Prostate Cancer, 5th edition (2019)
(French version: *Le cancer de la prostate*)

Jean Daniel Arbour, MD, Pierre Labelle, MD
and Florian Sennlaub, MD
AMD – Age-Related Macular Degeneration, 2nd edition (2016)
(French version: *DMLA – La dégénérescence maculaire liée à l'âge*, 2ᵉ édition)

Jean Daniel Arbour, MD, and Pierre Labelle, MD
Diabetic Retinopathy, 2nd edition (2016)
(French version: *La rétinopathie diabétique*)

Pierre Blondeau, MD, and Paul Harasymowycz, MD
Glaucoma (2014)
(French version: *Le glaucome*)

Fred Saad, MD, and Michael McCormack, MD
Prostate Diseases, 2nd edition (2013)
(French version: *Les maladies de la prostate*)

Fadi Massoud, MD, and Alain Robillard, MD
La maladie d'Alzheimer (2013)

WARNING
The content of this book is provided for information purposes only and cannot substitute for a consultation or the personalized advice of a doctor. We recommend that readers speak to a healthcare professional before beginning any treatment.

PROSTATE
CANCER

Fred Saad, MD

Michael McCormack, MD

Preface by Armen G. Aprikian, MD

Foreword by Dafydd Rhys Williams, MD, Astronaut

Fifth edition, entirely revised and updated, 2019

AP Annika Parance Publishing

AP Annika Parance Publishing
1043 Marie-Anne East
Montreal, Quebec H2J 2B5
514 658 7217
apediteur.com

English revision: Debby Dubrofsky
Book and cover design: Francis Desrosiers in collaboration with Scalpel Design
Layout: Ateliers Prêt-Presse

Bibliothèque et Archives nationales du Québec and Library and Archives Canada cataloguing in publication

Saad, Fred

    [Cancer de la prostate. English]

    Prostate cancer / Fred Saad, Michael McCormack.

    5th edition entirely revised.

    (Understand the disease and its treatment)
    Translation of : Le cancer de la prostate.
    Issued in print and electronic formats.

    ISBN 978-2-923830-75-9 (softcover)
    ISBN 978-2-923830-76-6 (PDF)
    ISBN 978-2-923830-77-3 (EPUB)

    1. Prostate - Cancer - Popular works. 2. Prostate - Cancer - Treatment - Popular works. I. McCormack, Michael, 1953-, author. II. Title. III. Title : Cancer de la prostate. English. IV. Series : Understand the disease and its treatment.

RC280.P7S2213 2018   616.99'463   C2018-942713-2
                                                                                                                         C2018-942714-0

Annika Parance Publishing acknowledges the financial support of the Government of Canada through the Canada Book Fund for its publishing activities.
Canadä

DISTRIBUTION OF ENGLISH TITLES IN CANADA AND THE USA	DISTRIBUTION OF FRENCH TITLES IN CANADA	DISTRIBUTION OF FRENCH TITLES IN EUROPE
Dimedia	Fitzhenry and Whiteside	Librairie du Québec (DNM)
Saint-Laurent (Québec)	Markham, Ontario	Paris
514-336-3941	1-800-387-9776	+33 (0) 1 43 54 49 02

Legal deposit – Bibliothèque et Archives nationales du Québec, 2019
Legal deposit – Library and Archives Canada, 2019

© Fred Saad and Michael McCormack, 2019
Annika Parance Publishing

All rights reserved.

Printed in Canada.

This book is dedicated to my patients, who show me how precious life is and make me feel useful in their fight against prostate cancer. It is also dedicated to my children, Geneviève, Julien, Véronique and Simon, and to my wonderful wife Rachel. I am grateful to them for accepting all the time I spend working on prostate cancer.

Dr. Fred Saad

This book is dedicated to men with prostate cancer and their families. It is also dedicated to my children Alie, Sophie and Marie-Hélène, and to my most wonderful wife Marie-Claude. I thank them for their support and encouragement in the pursuit of my academic activities.

Dr. Michael McCormack

The authors would also like to thank their publisher, Annika Parance for her excellent work.

Annika Parance Publishing would like to thank Dr. Françoise Le Deist for her invaluable assistance with this fifth edition and her insightful and knowledgeable contributions.

CONTENTS

THE AUTHORS 17
PREFACE 21
FOREWORD 23

25 FREQUENTLY ASKED QUESTIONS   25

CHAPTER 1
UNDERSTANDING PROSTATE CANCER   33

WHAT IS PROSTATE CANCER? 34
ANATOMY OF THE PROSTATE 36
FUNCTIONS OF THE PROSTATE 36
COMMON PROSTATE DISEASES 38
Benign prostatic hyperplasia 38
Prostatitis 39

PROSTATE CANCER INCIDENCE AND MORTALITY RATES IN CANADA 40

CHAPTER 2
RISK FACTORS   43

AGE 44
FAMILY HISTORY 44
GENES 45
RACE, POPULATIONS AND LIVING ENVIRONMENTS 45
NUTRITION 46
Consumption of animal fats and red meat 46
Calcium surplus and vitamin D deficiency 47
CHRONIC INFLAMMATION AND INFECTION 49
MALE HORMONES 49
KEY POINTS TO REMEMBER 52

CHAPTER 3
DIAGNOSIS   53

SYMPTOMS OF PROSTATE CANCER 54
SIGNS OF PROSTATE CANCER AND THE PHYSICAL EXAMINATION 56
PROSTATE SPECIFIC ANTIGEN (PSA) AND THE PSA TEST 57
TRANSRECTAL ULTRASOUND (TRUS) AND PROSTATE BIOPSY 60
Transrectal ultrasound (TRUS) 61
Prostate biopsy 62

ADDITIONAL TESTS 63
Lymphadenectomy 63
Bone scan 64
CT scan 64
Multiparametric magnetic resonance imaging (mpMRI) 64
Fusion biopsies 66
Prostate-specific membrane antigen positron emission
tomography (PSMA-PET) 67
CLASSIFICATION OF PROSTATE CANCER 67
Grading 68
Staging 70
KEY POINTS TO REMEMBER 73

CHAPTER 4
TREATMENT OF LOCALIZED PROSTATE CANCER — 77

SELECTING A TREATMENT 78
THE PATIENT'S OPTIONS 79
Men with a life expectancy of more than 10 years 81
Men with a life expectancy of less than 10 years 82
WATCHFUL WAITING AND ACTIVE SURVEILLANCE 85
Watchful waiting 85
Active surveillance 85
**RADICAL PROSTATECTOMY
(REMOVAL OF THE PROSTATE GLAND)** 86
Surgical techniques 89
    Open surgery 89
    Laparoscopic prostatectomy 90
    Robotic surgery 90
    Which technique is best? 90

Short-term complications of radical prostatectomy 92
Long-term complications of radical prostatectomy 93
Reducing the risk of complications of radical
prostatectomy 95
Results and medical follow-up of radical prostatectomy 96

RADIATION THERAPY 99
External beam radiation therapy 99
    Side effects of external beam radiation therapy 100
    Long-term complications of external beam
    radiation therapy 102
    Results and medical follow-up of external
    beam radiation therapy 103
Brachytherapy (permanent or temporary
radioactive implant) 104
    Side effects of brachytherapy 107
    Long-term complications of brachytherapy 107
    Results and medical follow-up of brachytherapy 108

FOCAL THERAPY 111
High-intensity focused ultrasound (HIFU) 111
Cryotherapy 111

HORMONE THERAPY 112
Side effects of hormone therapy 113
Long-term complications of hormone therapy 114
Results and medical follow-up of hormone therapy 114

PREDICTIVE TOOLS 115
Partin tables 115
Kattan nomograms 118
Albertsen life tables 118

KEY POINTS TO REMEMBER 120

CHAPTER 5
TREATMENT OF ADVANCED
PROSTATE CANCER — 123

HORMONE THERAPY 124
Orchiectomy (surgical castration) 124
LH-RH analog therapy (medical castration) 126
Side effects of hormone therapy 128
Long-term complications of hormone therapy 129
Medical follow-up of hormone therapy 131

**RECURRENCE AFTER TREATMENT
OF LOCALIZED CANCER** 131
Recurrence after radical prostatectomy 132
Recurrence after radiation therapy
(external or brachytherapy) 133

LOCALLY ADVANCED NON-METASTATIC CANCER 134

METASTATIC CANCER 135
Nodal metastasis 135
Bone metastasis 135

WHEN HORMONE THERAPY IS NOT ENOUGH 136
Castration-resistant prostate cancer (CRPC)
with detectable metastasis 137
    Chemotherapy 137
        Docetaxel (Taxotere) 137
            Men with metastasis at diagnosis 138
            Side effects of docetaxel 139
        Treatment options after docetaxel 140
            Cabazitaxel (Jevtana) 140
    New generation hormone therapy 141
        Abiraterone (Zytiga) 141
        Enzalutamide (Xtandi) 142
    Managing bone metastasis 143
        Radium 223 (Xofigo) 143

Side effects of radium-223 143
Results and medical monitoring with radium-223 144
Bone-targeted supportive therapy 144
Castration-resistant prostate cancer (CRPC) without
detectable metastasis 145
SUMMARY 146

CHAPTER 6
LIVING WITH PROSTATE CANCER — 149

SUPPORT FROM THE DOCTOR 150
MEDICAL FOLLOW-UP 152
SEX 154
Oral treatments for erectile dysfunction 155
Other solutions 156
    Urethral suppository (or Muse) 156
    Intracavernous injection 157
    Vacuum pump (or external pump) 158
    Penile implants 159
    Alternative solutions 161
SUPPORT FROM THE FAMILY 161
PROFESSIONAL PSYCHOSOCIAL SUPPORT 163
OTHER SOURCES OF SUPPORT 165

CHAPTER 7
NUTRITIONAL GUIDE — 167

EPIDEMIOLOGY OF PROSTATE CANCER 168
DIETARY FAT 170
VITAMIN E 171

SELENIUM	172
LYCOPENE	173
SOY PROTEIN	173
GREEN TEA	174
INSULIN RESISTANCE	174
FLAX SEED	175
VITAMIN D	175
KEY POINTS TO REMEMBER	176
USEFUL ADDRESSES	177
GLOSSARY	183

LIST OF BOXES

Myths and realities	35
What the prostate doesn't do	39
Canadian cancer society statistics	40
Age-standardized incidence and mortality rates for the most common cancers in men	41
Incidence, mortality, lifetime probability and survival statistics for selected cancers, in men	42
Prostate, breast and ovarian cancer: is there a link?	44
What are free radicals?	47
Vitamin D supplement	48
Nobel prize for male hormone research	50
Key points to remember from chapter 2	52
Prostate cancer screening recommendations	55
Age- and race-specific upper limits of normal for PSA	58
The pathologist	62

Grading and staging of prostate cancer 72
Key points to remember from chapter 3 73
Questions to ask the doctor 80
Pre-operative procedures 88
Cancer in older men is still serious 99
Does the penis really get smaller? 102
High-dose rate (HDR) brachytherapy 109
Key points to remember from chapter 4 120
LH-RH analogs 127
Anti-androgens 128
Continuous or intermittent LH-RH analog therapy? 130
Chemotherapy (not as bad as it sounds!) 140
It's still possible to start a family 151
Who does what? 153
A sex therapist can often be helpful 160
Being ill shouldn't mean giving up 162
Overcoming shyness and pride 164
Key points to remember rom chapter 7 176

THE AUTHORS

Fred Saad, MD
Dr. Fred Saad is a professor of surgery at the University of Montréal. He is currently chief of urology and director of urologic oncology at the University of Montréal Hospital Centre (*Centre Hospitalier de l'Université de Montréal, CHUM*). He also heads the Molecular Prostate Cancer Research Lab at the Montréal Cancer Institute and is director of oncology research at the CHUM research centre. Since 2004, he has held the Raymond Garneau Chair in Prostate Cancer Research.

Dr. Saad is president of the Canadian Urologic Association and is past president of the Québec Urological Association and of the National Cancer Institute of Canada G-U Group. He is a member of ten editorial boards and serves as a reviewer for more than 30 urology and oncology journals. He has published over 500 scientific articles and book chapters and has collaborated on over 1500 scientific abstracts presented at meetings around the world. He is co-editor of several books, including *Prostate Cancer*, which has sold over 200,000 copies since the first edition was published in 2004.

His main research interests include molecular prognostic markers in prostate cancer and new treatments for advanced prostate cancer. He is currently coordinating more than 40 clinical and basic research projects in urologic oncology. Nationally and internationally, he has been a guest speaker or lecturer over 400 times, thanks to his involvement in research and medical education. In 2005, he received the CHUM Leadership Award in Medicine, and in 2014 he received the CHUM research centre's lifetime achievement award. In 2018 he received the highest honor given by the Québec government, the National Order of Québec, for his contributions to the field of prostate cancer.

Michael McCormack, MD
Dr. Michael McCormack is a urologist, the assistant head of urology at the University of Montréal Hospital Centre (*Centre Hospitalier de l'Université de Montréal, CHUM*) and clinical professor in the Department of Surgery, Faculty of Medicine, University of Montréal.

After completing his studies in medullary neurophysiology at McGill University, Dr. McCormack studied medicine at the University of Montréal. He received his medical doctorate in 1983 and finished his urology training in 1988. He chose to begin his career in private practice in Saint-Jean-sur-Richelieu, where he was also head of urology service and head of the surgery department at the regional hospital. In 2000, he joined the urology team at CHUM.

Dr. McCormack served as chair of the Québec college of physicians' urology examination committee and vice-chair of the Examination Board in Urology at the Royal College of Physicians and Surgeons of Canada. He has chaired the IT Committee of the Canadian Urological Association and was an associate editor for the Canadian Urological Association Journal. He is a past president of the Québec Urological Association and is currently responsible for the evaluation and teaching of residents in urologic surgery at CHUM.

Dr. McCormack has contributed several chapters to medical books and is the author of two books on medical topics for the general public: *Male Sexual Health* (2003) and *Prostate Cancer*, which he co-authored and which has sold over 200,000 copies since the first edition was published in 2004.

In 2010, Dr. McCormack was awarded a Prix Esculape in recognition of the excellence of his teaching at CHUM.

SPECIAL CONTRIBUTORS TO CHAPTER 4, TREATMENT OF LOCALIZED PROSTATE CANCER

Guila Delouya, MD
Radiation Oncologist, Department of Radiation Oncology and Nuclear Medicine, University of Montréal Hospital Centre (CHUM)
Associate Clinical Professor, Faculty of Medicine, University of Montréal

Daniel Taussky, MD
Radiation Oncologist, Department of Radiation Oncology, University of Montréal Hospital Centre (CHUM)

Louise Lambert, MD
Radiation Oncologist, Department of Radiation Oncology, University of Montréal Hospital Centre (CHUM)

Frédéric Arsenault, MD
Nuclear Radiologist, Department of Radiology, Radiation Oncology and Nuclear Medicine, University of Montréal Hospital Centre (CHUM)

SPECIAL CONTRIBUTORS TO CHAPTER 6, LIVING WITH PROSTATE CANCER

Luc Valiquette, MD
Urologist, University of Montréal Hospital Centre (CHUM)
Professor, Department of Surgery, Faculty of Medicine, University of Montréal

Claudie Giguère, PhD
Oncology Psychologist, Service of Psychology, University of Montréal Hospital Centre (CHUM)

Renée Pichette, MA
Clinical Sexologist and Oncology Psychotherapist, Service of Psychology, University of Montréal Hospital Centre (CHUM)

SPECIAL CONTRIBUTOR TO CHAPTER 7, NUTRITIONAL GUIDE

Neil Eric Fleshner, MD
Urologist and Love Chair in Prostate Cancer Prevention, Princess Margaret Hospital, University Health Network
Chief, division of Urology, University of Toronto

PREFACE

Prostate cancer is the most frequently diagnosed cancer in men today, and the third leading cause of death from cancer in Canada.

As a urologic oncologist who treats men with prostate cancer and helps their families deal with the disease, I am often asked for literature to help with the myriad of issues patients face. Although several helpful books are available, this work by Dr. Fred Saad and Dr. Michael McCormack is among the most useful I have come across, and I regularly offer it to my patients.

The key to any medical book dealing with a complex topic like prostate cancer is the ability to explain the issues clearly, concisely and comprehensively. I believe the authors of this book have succeeded in providing men and their families with all the information they require to help them through the difficult times during their illness.

Men are often so shaken when they are first told they have prostate cancer that they cannot focus on all the other important information their doctor is telling them. They leave the consultation room feeling terrified, still troubled by a number of questions they wish they had asked. This book can help allay some of their fears and answer many of their questions. More importantly, it can help them prepare the right questions to ask their doctors during subsequent consultations.

This 5th edition is well written, easy to read and superbly illustrated. Importantly, it provides an in-depth update on new treatments that have become available in recent years and are prolonging the lives of men with prostate cancer. It continues to provide the latest medical information, spanning the disease spectrum from prevention and diagnosis to treatment and palliative care. The book also explains the potential side effects and consequences of the different treatments on a man's quality of life. Finally, it is one of the few books that devotes considerable attention to the significant psychological impact of a prostate cancer diagnosis on an individual and his loved ones.

I applaud Dr. Saad and Dr. McCormack for updating this wonderful book. I am confident it will help numerous men and their families as they cope with prostate cancer. The more men know about prostate cancer, the more they will be able to help themselves and meet the disease head on.

Armen G. Aprikian, MD
Director, Cancer Care Mission
McGill University Hospital Centre (MUHC)
Richard Tomlinson Chair for Urology Research
Professor, Department of Surgery/Urology
McGill University

FOREWORD

"You have prostate cancer." Four words no one ever wants to hear, yet one in seven Canadian men will develop prostate cancer during their lifetime! And though most men are over 60 when diagnosed, many are in their forties or fifties.

Like other forms of cancer, this disease affects not only the patient but also his spouse and family. There are so many questions when a man is first diagnosed with prostate cancer, yet before the publication of this book there was no single work that explained prostate cancer simply and concisely and could serve as a guide for patients recently diagnosed or undergoing treatment and their families. This volume is an outstanding source of information on the prevention, causes and early diagnosis of prostate cancer and the current treatment options, including their side effects and complications.

In addition, this book tackles topics that are often overlooked, such as the psychological impact of the disease and the effect of its treatment on sexual function and virility. The numerous options available to help men preserve their virility are discussed, and the many stories of men with the disease who continue to lead happy and productive lives for years offer reassurance. The book also looks at the role of diet and nutritional supplements in the prevention of prostate cancer, making it a valuable resource for men with an increased risk of developing the disease.

Though the incidence of prostate cancer is on the rise, recent advances in treatment have led to a decrease in the risk of death, and impressive advances in minimally invasive surgery that can treat certain forms of the disease mean fewer complications and more rapid recovery. While a diagnosis of prostate cancer is still devastating news, the impact is now very different from what it was in the past. Though we still have much to learn about prostate cancer, there is a tremendous amount of active research taking place all over the world, giving us very good reason to believe that the quality of life of men with prostate cancer will continue to improve in the years ahead.

Dafydd Rhys Williams, MD
Astronaut, Canadian Space Agency
Prostate cancer survivor

25 FREQUENTLY ASKED QUESTIONS

(1) What is cancer?

Cancer is characterized by uncontrolled growth of abnormal cells. After a while, groups of these cells form a detectable lesion (or lump) known as a tumour (cancer). Cancer can affect any type of cell in an organ, a gland, muscle tissue, blood or the lymphatic system. In the case of prostate cancer, the secretory cells are usually the ones that become cancerous. In theory, there are two types of prostate cancer: slow-growing and aggressive. In reality, most cases are somewhere between the two, growing at a moderate rate. For the moment, scientists do not have the tools to accurately predict the growth rate of a person's cancer once it has been diagnosed (Chapter 1).

(2) What is metastasis?

Over time, the malignant cells in cancerous tumours can invade neighbouring tissue or organs. They may even spread to the rest of the body through the blood or lymphatic system. The presence of prostate cancer cells anywhere outside the prostate is called metastasis. The most common sites of metastases in prostate cancer are lymph nodes and bones (Chapters 1 and 4).

③ Is prostate cancer very common?

Yes. Prostate cancer is the most common cancer among Canadian men (excluding non-melanoma skin cancer). In 2017, according to the Canadian Cancer Society, an estimated 21,300 Canadian men were diagnosed with prostate cancer and 4,100 died of it. Every day, on average, 58 Canadian men are diagnosed with prostate cancer and 11 die of it. One in seven men will develop prostate cancer during his lifetime (the risk increases with age) and one in 29 will die of it (Chapter 1).

④ What are the symptoms?

Most prostate cancers develop without symptoms, and those affected are frequently completely unaware they have the disease until it is detected by a doctor. In fact, 80 percent of prostate cancer cases are discovered during routine medical checkups. Furthermore, those affected may feel perfectly healthy and be symptom-free regardless of the stage of the disease when detected (Chapter 3).

⑤ What is the difference between benign prostatic hypertrophy (BPH) and prostate cancer?

BPH is a benign growth of the prostate. Why the prostate grows and eventually blocks the passage of urine is unclear but is considered a normal consequence of aging. As opposed to prostate cancer, the cells that grow and multiply are normal in every way and there is no risk of spread to other parts of the body. BPH does not require treatment unless symptoms are bothersome (Chapter 1).

(6) What are the risk factors for prostate cancer?

Our knowledge of prostate cancer is currently incomplete, particularly when it comes to risk factors. Age and family history of prostate cancer are the most important risk factors. Diet and other environmental factors may also contribute. Most men diagnosed with prostate cancer are over 60 years of age (Chapter 2).

(7) Is prostate cancer hereditary?

Men with a family history of prostate cancer run a higher risk of developing the disease and are more likely to do so at a younger age. A man whose father or brother had prostate cancer is twice as likely to suffer from the disease as someone with no family history. If two relatives had it (for example, father and a brother or two brothers), the risk is even greater. It has been determined that a familial or hereditary predisposition is found in only about 15 percent of prostate cancer cases. It appears likely that both genetics and the environment play a role in the development of prostate cancer (Chapter 2).

(8) Can prostate cancer be prevented?

It is possible that alterations in dietary intake, coupled with the consumption of certain micronutrients, may have an impact on prostate cancer. For now nothing is proven and approved for the prevention of prostate cancer (Chapter 7).

(9) Who can treat prostate cancer?

Urologists and radiation oncologists usually treat prostate cancer when first diagnosed. In the case of metastasis, and especially when chemotherapy is involved, medical oncologists often become part of the team. In addition, the patient's healthcare team (including family doctors, nurses, radiation oncology technologists and volunteers) is there to offer comfort and support (Chapters 3 and 4).

⑩ What types of medical tests are involved? Are they painful?

A combination of three tests help detect prostate cancer: digital rectal exam (DRE), PSA blood test and prostate biopsy. The DRE involves the doctor inserting a gloved finger into the patient's rectum and palpating the gland. In its normal state, the prostate is smooth and rubbery. The doctor therefore checks for a lump or induration (hardening). Although useful, the DRE is by no means a perfect diagnostic test since it is not possible to examine the entire prostate. Most cases of prostate cancer diagnosed in Canada are not detected through a physical examination but with the help of PSA testing. To determine whether cancer is present requires a biopsy that is done with the guidance of an ultrasound probe placed in the rectum. This is a little painful but necessary to make the diagnosis of prostate cancer. It is only done when the DRE or PSA is abnormal (Chapter 3).

⑪ What is PSA?

Prostate specific antigen (PSA) is a glycoprotein (a protein mixed with a molecule of sugar) produced by normal prostate cells. A certain amount of PSA is also found in the bloodstream.

The levels of PSA may vary according to age and race. The more cells there are in the prostate, the more PSA is produced; therefore, the concentration is naturally higher in men over the age of 40 because of the increased size of the gland, even if there is no cancer. In cases of cancer, more PSA may leak into the blood and therefore, in most patients, levels are higher (Chapter 3).

⑫ Is it possible to have prostate cancer despite a normal PSA level?

Yes. PSA levels can be considered normal (below 4) in patients who have the disease. According to a study published in 2004 in the New England Journal of Medicine, PSA concentrations remain "normal" in 15 percent of men who have the disease. This result is known as a "false negative" PSA value (Chapter 3).

⑬ Does a high PSA level always mean prostate cancer?

No. Elevated PSA levels indicate a prostate condition, but not necessarily prostate cancer. In addition to age, race and benign prostatic hyperplasia, the possible causes of high PSA levels include inflammation of the prostate and urinary tract infection. In most cases, levels return to normal once the problem is treated. Any trauma to the prostate (biopsy, surgery, etc) can also cause a temporary increase in PSA, leading to what is known as a "false positive" result. It is therefore very important not to jump to conclusions. It should be noted, however, that a digital rectal exam (DRE) very rarely causes such an elevation (Chapter 3).

⑭ Does sexual activity affect the PSA level?

Not in any significant manner.

⑮ If the cancer is caught at an early stage what are the options?

If the cancer is localized and limited to the prostate, cure is very likely and patients will have choices. Treatment will depend on the aggressivity of the cancer and on the patient's age, life expectancy and preference. Options may include active surveillance or treatment with surgery or radiation therapy (Chapter 4).

16 **If the cancer is found in only one side of the prostate, is it possible to remove only the cancerous part?**
No. Even though a digital rectal examination or a prostate biopsy may show cancer on only one side, prostate cancer is often a multi-focal disease and multiple sites of cancer are generally found throughout the prostate. This is why it is essential to remove the entire prostate in the case of surgery and to treat the entire prostate in the case of external beam radiation therapy or brachytherapy (Chapter 4).

17 **Is it possible to predict how aggressive the cancer is and the chances of a cure?**
Doctors cannot precisely predict exactly how aggressive a newly diagnosed cancer is or the risk of progression, although they do have some tools to help guide the patient, namely the Partin tables, the Kattan nomograms and the Albertsen life tables. These tools may help predict the risk the cancer poses for the patient (Chapter 4).

18 **Can prostate cancer go away by itself?**
No, but some prostate cancers may progress very slowly. They can be present for years and never spread, produce symptoms or threaten the life of the patient. Older men (generally those over the age of 70) with slow-growing cancer may very likely die of another condition before the cancer becomes a threat. When all signs indicate the cancer is slow-growing, the selected course of action may be to wait for symptoms to appear before beginning treatment. It is important in certain cases to weigh the inconvenience of treatment with the risk posed by the cancer (Chapter 4).

19 **Are all patients affected by side effects of treatments?**
Treatment for prostate cancer generally leads to some degree of sexual dysfunction (which is usually treatable); however, libido and orgasms are preserved unless hormone

therapy is given. Urinary incontinence is infrequent and is usually due to surgery. Radiation therapy may lead to rectal and bladder irritation. Hormone therapy generally leads to loss of libido and sexual problems as well as hot flashes (Chapters 4 and 5).

(20) My PSA is going up and I had a treatment that was supposed to cure me. What happened?
When PSA rises after treatment of any kind, this usually indicates the cancer has come back. Unfortunately, no treatment can guarantee a cure. Depending on how aggressive the cancer was at the time of diagnosis, the risk the cancer will recur will vary. PSA testing allows the doctor to detect the recurrence of prostate cancer early and may allow for additional treatment to control the disease before it has spread to other organs (Chapters 3 and 4).

(21) If the cancer has already spread to the bones, is there any treatment?
Yes. There is hope, even at the latest stage of prostate cancer. Even though cure is not possible, with hormone therapy patients may live for years with a very good quality of life. Research continues to improve patients' life expectancy and quality of life (Chapter 5).

(22) The cancer is progressing even on hormone therapy. Is there any hope?
This has been the biggest area of research over the last 10 years, and many new treatments have become available that help prolong men's lives and quality of life. Chemotherapy and newer forms of hormone therapy are keeping patients alive and well longer. Other treatments are available to help strengthen bones and reduce the risks of complications from cancer that has spread there. We are also seeing

the emergence of new options, including exciting treatments that are still under investigation (Chapter 5).

23 Is it possible to be cured of prostate cancer?
Yes. If the cancer is caught early, remains confined to the prostate and is treated in a timely manner, it can generally be cured (Chapter 4).

24 Must I take food supplements?
Because of our northern latitude, the sun's rays are weaker in the fall and winter. We therefore recommend that Canadian adults consider taking a vitamin D supplement. Talk to your doctor about taking 1000 international units (IU) a day during fall and winter months (Chapters 2 and 7).

25 I have been asked to participate in a clinical trial (protocol). Should I do it?
Research enables us to improve the way we treat cancer. Our understanding of cancer and all the new treatments we now have are due to research that involved men with prostate cancer. By participating in a clinical trial, you could have access to new therapies. A trial entails close follow-up to determine how effective the new treatment is compared to the standard therapy (if there is one) and to identify side effects. In the vast majority of cases, the advantages of being part of a clinical trial are much greater than the disadvantages. Patients who are interested should always ask their doctor about any ongoing studies that may be of benefit to them.

CHAPTER 1
UNDERSTANDING PROSTATE CANCER

The verdict is in: "It's prostate cancer." For the man receiving this diagnosis, two worrying questions immediately spring to mind: "Can it be cured?" and "Will it affect my virility?" Although these concerns are perfectly normal, most patients usually find their anxiety eases once treatment starts and they begin to understand their illness better.

Prostate cancer is curable if diagnosed in the early stages. If the disease is more advanced, treatment can ease the symptoms and prolong life. It is also worth pointing out that prostate cancer rarely causes erectile dysfunction—which is usually brought about by some of the treatments for the disease, not the disease itself.

There are various causes and forms of prostate cancer. The evolution of the disease can vary significantly from one person to the next. Although scientific knowledge has become much more precise over the last 20 years, many aspects of this insidious disease remain a mystery. Happily, however, the treatments available have improved considerably in recent years, meaning a greater number of men can continue to lead long and productive lives.

WHAT IS PROSTATE CANCER?

Generally speaking, cancer is characterized by uncontrolled growth of abnormal cells. It can affect any type of cell in an organ, a gland, muscle tissue, blood or the lymphatic system.

Under normal conditions, the cells in our bodies contain all the information they need for their development, function, reproduction and death. Usually, our cells do their work properly and we remain healthy. However, sometimes a few of the cells do not behave normally and begin multiplying uncontrollably, eventually forming a group of abnormal cells. After a while, this group forms a detectable lump known as a tumour.

Over time, the malignant cells in cancerous tumours can invade neighbouring tissue or organs. They may even spread to the rest of the body through the blood or lymphatic system. This stage is known as "metastasis."

In the case of prostate cancer, the secretory cells are usually the ones that become cancerous. Once the cancer has been diagnosed, treatment is determined depending on the stage of the disease and the overall health of the patient.

In theory, there are two types of prostate cancer: slow-growing and aggressive. In reality, most cases are somewhere between the two, growing at a moderate rate. For the moment, science does not have the tools to predict the growth rate of a person's cancer once it has been diagnosed.

About 14 percent of Canadians suffer from "clinical" prostate cancer, meaning their disease has been detected by a doctor and officially diagnosed. However, studies of autopsy reports have shown that another 30 percent of men have latent cancer, meaning the cancerous cells lie dormant in the prostate. Although present, the cancer does no harm because it does not attack the body. Not all men develop latent prostate cancer, but the probability of doing so increases with age.

According to the current state of knowledge, prostate cancer is one of the few cancers that can remain in latent form for such a long period of time. Researchers are trying to understand why some cancers remain latent while others develop into full-blown diseases. While it is generally believed that risk factors and genes play an important role in the development of clinically significant cancer, the precise mechanism is still unknown.

MYTHS AND REALITIES

I have urinary problems, so I probably have prostate cancer.
Myth. The vast majority of patients who have trouble emptying their bladders (a condition known as lower urinary tract symptoms (LUTS) or prostatism) are not suffering from prostate cancer, but rather from benign prostatic hyperplasia.

Erectile dysfunction is a sign of prostate cancer.
Myth. Prostate cancer rarely causes erectile problems. However, the treatments for the disease might.

Prostate cancer is not fatal.
Myth. Many newly diagnosed men shrug their shoulders and say, "It could be worse. At least it's not fatal." But they're wrong. Although more men die of cardiovascular disease and lung cancer, prostate cancer is still a significant cause of death in Canada.

ANATOMY OF THE PROSTATE

The prostate is a gland that produces the fluid necessary to carry semen during ejaculation. When healthy, it is about the size of a walnut and weighs no more than 20 grams. It is located under the bladder and surrounds the urethra, the canal that transports urine out of the body. The prostate is also next to the seminal vesicles. Because the back of the gland touches the rectum, a doctor can assess its size and consistency by performing a digital rectal exam (Figure ❶).

The prostate of a young boy is tiny. During puberty, when the voice changes and body hair begins to develop, the prostate gland, penis, testicles and scrotum also begin to grow due to an increase in the levels of testosterone (a male sex hormone).

The prostate is considered one of the male reproductive organs because it secretes nutrients and liquid for sperm cells, ensuring their survival. The prostate is therefore most "useful" to a man when he decides to start a family.

FUNCTIONS OF THE PROSTATE

In the average ejaculate (the contents of one ejaculation), there are between twenty and one hundred million spermatozoa (or sperm cells). However, sperm cells still account for only one to five percent of the total volume of semen. The substances that make up the rest are produced mainly by the prostate and seminal vesicles, and they are mixed together just before ejaculation.

Some of these substances (proteins and zinc) protect against bacteria and reduce the acidity of vaginal secretions so the sperm cells are not destroyed. Semen also contains amino acids and large quantities of fructose (a sugar) that provide energy to the sperm cells, as well as prostaglandins which, once in the vagina, trigger muscle contractions that push semen farther back into the uterus.

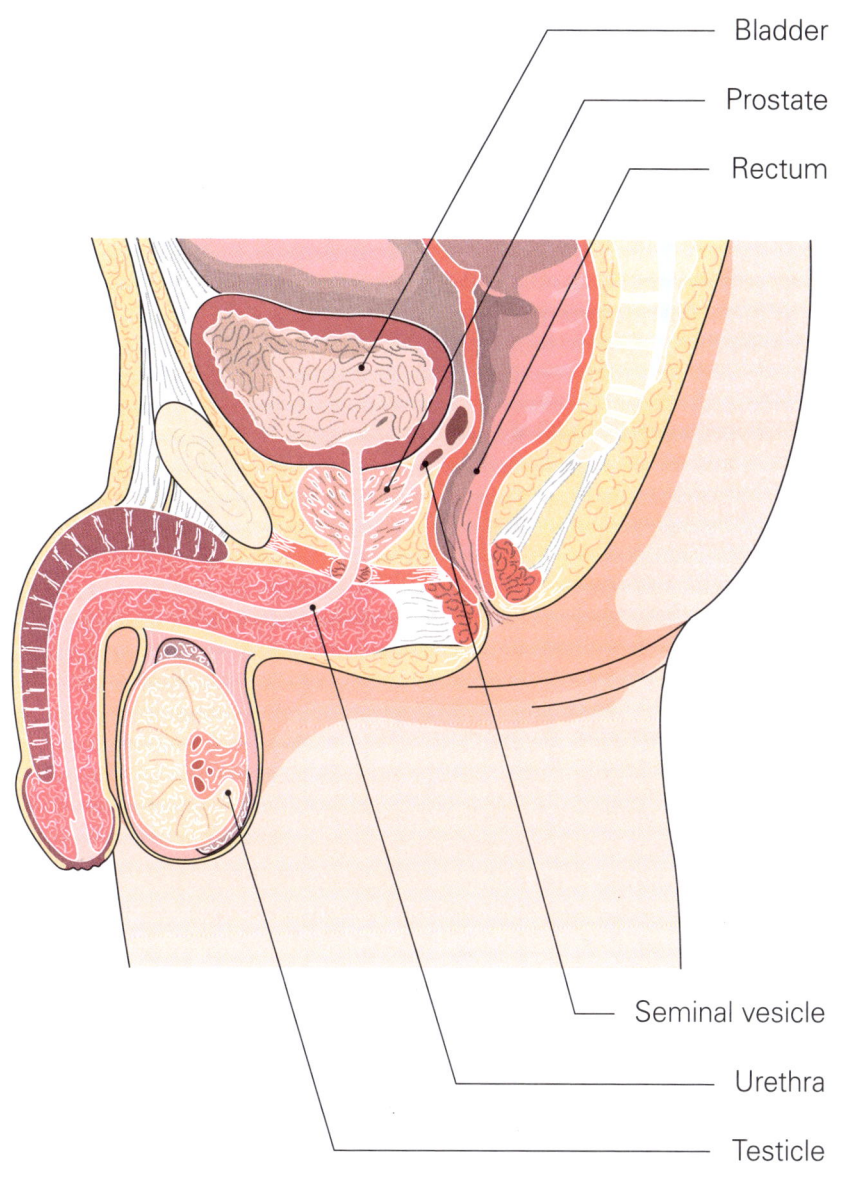

❶ Anatomy of the prostate and the surrounding organs

The prostate also produces a protein called prostate-specific antigen (PSA). It is generally believed that PSA helps liquefy semen and that this plays a role in fertility.

Put simply, the prostate contributes to male fertility by secreting substances that are essential to creating an environment in which sperm cells can survive. Without the prostate, "natural" fertilization is impossible.

Furthermore, the prostate is composed not only of secretory (also called exocrine) cells but also of muscle cells that help evacuate the sperm during ejaculation.

COMMON PROSTATE DISEASES

Trouble urinating may lead men to believe they have prostate cancer. However, while it is true that this is one of the symptoms of the disease, non-cancerous prostate diseases are most often the cause of urinary problems and are more common than cancer. A doctor should be consulted for a clear diagnosis.

Benign prostatic hyperplasia

After the age of 30, the prostate begins to enlarge slowly. This phenomenon is still not completely understood, although testosterone is known to be a contributing factor. Because it surrounds the urinary canal, the gland can block the passage of liquid through this canal as it enlarges, leading to various possible symptoms, such as difficulty urinating, reduced urine stream, inability to completely empty the bladder, constant need to urinate, or urine leaking or dripping. These obstructive and irritative symptoms are known as lower urinary tract symptoms (LUTS) or prostatism.

Although unpleasant, benign prostatic hyperplasia is non-cancerous. In fact, it is a common disorder that affects nearly all men as they age (about 25 percent require treatment). A doctor can prescribe medication to ease the symptoms; in more serious cases, surgery may be required to remove the part of the prostate that is causing the obstruction.

Prostatitis

Infectious prostatitis can be caused by bacteria from a urinary or sexually transmitted infection. This acute disease generally causes the following symptoms: high fever, chills, lower abdominal pain, back pain, frequent need to urinate, burning during urination and ejaculation, and difficulty urinating or ejaculating. In some cases, there is blood in the semen. Antibiotic treatment will usually clear the infection.

Some men experience lower abdominal pain during urination or ejaculation even in the absence of infection. While this condition used to be called chronic prostatitis, it is now known in the medical community as chronic pelvic pain, since it is a disorder that is little understood and may not be related to the prostate. Treatment may take the form of antibiotics, anti-inflammatories or relaxants for the smooth muscles of the prostate.

WHAT THE PROSTATE DOESN'T DO

There is a persistent myth that the prostate is required for penile erection. This explains why so many men who experience erectile dysfunction (ED) become worried that they may be suffering from prostate disease. It is true that the nerves required for normal erections are placed quite close to the prostate. However, the prostate itself is not involved in the mechanism of erection. If a man is experiencing ED, he should look elsewhere for the cause.

PROSTATE CANCER INCIDENCE AND MORTALITY RATES IN CANADA

In Canada, the incidence of prostate cancer peaked in 1993 and again in 2001. Each of these peaks was followed by a decline. These peaks are compatible with two waves of intensified screening activity using the prostate-specific antigen (PSA) test. Since 2001, the incidence rate has generally been declining.

The mortality rate for prostate cancer has been declining since the late 1990s. The decline likely reflects a combination of earlier detection and improved treatment.

To find out more, consult the website of the Canadian Cancer Society at www.cancer.ca.

CANADIAN CANCER SOCIETY STATISTICS

Prostate cancer is the most common cancer among Canadian men (excluding non-melanoma skin cancer).

In 2017:

- An estimated 21,300 Canadian men were diagnosed with prostate cancer and 4,100 died of it.
- On average, 58 Canadian men were diagnosed with prostate cancer every day.
- On average, 11 Canadian men died of prostate cancer every day.
- One in 7 men will develop prostate cancer during his lifetime (the risk is highest after age 60) and one in 29 will die of it.

CHAPTER 1 – UNDERSTANDING PROSTATE CANCER

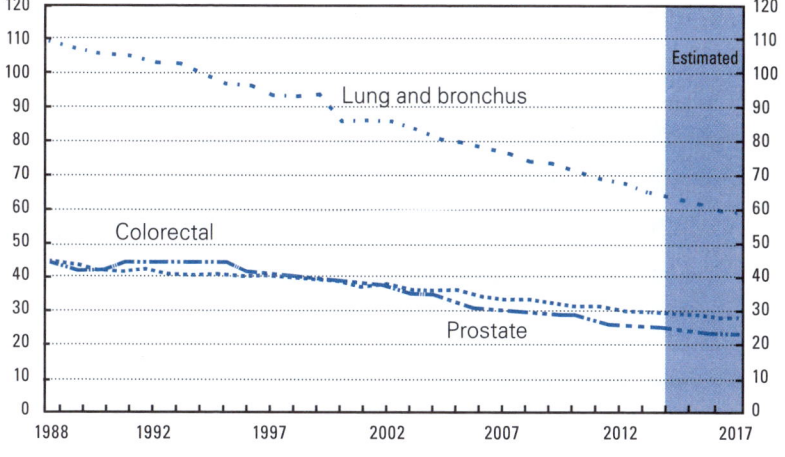

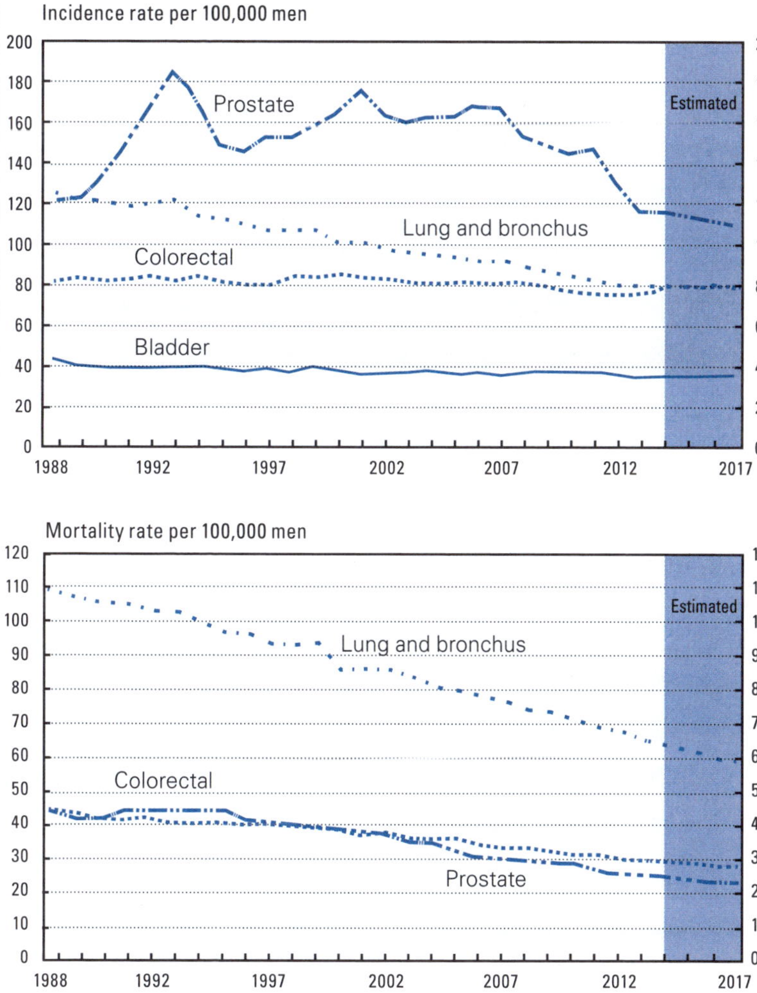

INCIDENCE, MORTALITY, LIFETIME PROBABILITY AND SURVIVAL STATISTICS FOR SELECTED CANCERS, IN MEN (CANADA, 2017)*

Males	Projected incidence		Projected mortality		Lifetime probability of developing and dying from cancer, respectively		5-year net survival
	Rank	Cases	Rank	Deaths	One in:	One in:	%
All cancers	—	103,100	—	42,600	2	3.5	60
Prostate	1	21,300	3	4,100	7	29	95
Colorectal	2	14,900	2	5,100	13	29	63
Lung and bronchus	3	14,400	1	11,100	11	14	14
Bladder	4	6,700	5	1,700	25	83	74
Non-Hodgkin lymphoma	5	4,600	8	1,500	43	95	63
Kidney and renal pelvis	6	4,200	11	1,200	54	142	66
Melanoma	7	4,000	15	790	56	241	85
Leukemia	8	3,600	6	1,650	51	90	58
Oral	9	3,200	13	860	68	206	60
Pancreas	10	2,800	4	2,400	74	72	7
Stomach	11	2,200	10	1,250	78	126	23
Liver	12	1,900	12	950	127	199	19
Esophagus	13	1,800	7	1,650	112	112	13
Brain/CNS	14,15	1,700	9	1,350	123	163	22
Multiple myeloma	14,15	1,700	14	810	117	179	42
Thyroid	16	1,650	17	95	189	1,512	95
Testis	17	1,100	20	45	247	—	96
Larynx	18	970	16	350	170	459	64
Hodgkin lymphoma	19	570	18	85	426	—	83
Breast	20	230	19	60	756	—	79
Other cancers	—	9,600	—	5,500	—	—	—

* Column totals may not sum to row totals due to rounding.
—: Fewer than three deaths

Source: Canadian Cancer Statistics Advisory Committee. *Canadian Cancer Statistics 2017.* Toronto, ON: Canadian Cancer Society; 2018. Available at: cancer.ca/Canadian-Cancer-Statistics-2018-EN

CHAPTER 2
RISK FACTORS

Our knowledge of prostate cancer is currently incomplete, particularly when it comes to risk factors. Our understanding is evolving, however, and the large number of studies now underway worldwide will surely lead to more clarity within the next few years. In the meantime, the following sections provide a useful overview of what we know today. It is worth noting that prostate cancer cannot be attributed to a single cause, and it sometimes presents in men with none of these risk factors.

AGE

Prostate cancer is associated with aging. It generally affects men over the age of 50, increasing in prevalence (number of cases) with age. It is very rare in men under 40 (less than one percent); when it does occur in this age group, it is usually due to genetic factors.

FAMILY HISTORY

Men with a family history of prostate cancer run a higher risk of developing the disease and are more likely to do so at a younger age. A man whose father or brother had prostate cancer is twice as likely to suffer from the disease as someone with no family history. If two relatives had it (for example, father and brother, two or more brothers, both grandfathers, two uncles, etc.), the risk is even greater. This is true whether the relatives are on the mother's or father's side. The risk increases even more if the close family members were diagnosed before the age of 50. That said, inherited or "familial" cancer is not "worse" than non-familial (also known as sporadic) cancer. The prognosis (risk of dying of the disease) is based much more on the stage, grade and PSA level at the time of diagnosis than on family history. If a man's cancer is familial, he should not assume

> **PROSTATE, BREAST AND OVARIAN CANCER: IS THERE A LINK?**
>
> Studies have indicated that men with relatives who had breast or ovarian cancer may run a higher risk of developing prostate cancer. While these results are quite interesting, they are also recent.

that his prognosis will be the same as his father's or grandfather's. The most important predictor of the outcome of the disease is the stage at which it is diagnosed. In other words, if a family member died of prostate cancer, early detection is crucial to improve the chances of a cure.

Both genetics and the environment play a role in the development of prostate cancer. It is thought that a familial or hereditary predisposition is a factor in only about 15 percent of prostate cancer cases

GENES

It is likely that genes play a role in prostate cancer, even in the 85 percent of cases that are non-hereditary. While the function of genes is not fully understood at present, researchers do know that they play a role in the development and progression of the disease. It is hoped that one day scientists will be able to create a genetic profile for the disease that will lead to more accurate screening and treatment methods.

RACE, POPULATIONS AND LIVING ENVIRONMENTS

The risk of developing prostate cancer seems to vary from population to population. The disease is much more common in the Western world, for example Canada, the United States, northern Europe and Australia. For reasons that are not well understood, African-American men have the highest rate in the world, with many developing the disease before the age of 50.

In contrast, prevalence is much lower in other parts of the world, such as Asia (Japan, China and Thailand), a number of North African countries and the Middle East. Men in Japan, for example, are ten times less likely to have prostate cancer than North American men; men in China are up to 100 times less likely to develop the disease than African-American men.

Can we therefore conclude that prostate cancer is associated with genetic racial characteristics? Not necessarily, since a person's living environment and lifestyle practices are also important factors. Scientists have noted, for example, that Japanese people who have been living in North America for at least one generation run the same risks as people born here, leading them to suspect that there is something about living in a "rich" industrialized country that leads to unhealthy lifestyle practices, particularly when it comes to eating habits. Indeed, diet is one of the risk factors being focused on extensively in prostate cancer research.

NUTRITION

Consumption of animal fats and red meat

The body needs dietary fat to function properly. However, a clear link has been established between fat consumption and the risk of prostate cancer. Several statistical studies have highlighted a significant correlation between consumption of animal fat and prostate cancer growth and mortality rates. Other studies have shown that a diet containing substantial amounts of red meat also increases the risk.

Scientists do not fully comprehend the exact mechanisms by which dietary fat can influence prostate cancer. Theories revolve around the effects fats have on hormones, the production of free radicals (see box, "What are free radicals?"), the low amounts of anti-carcinogenic ingredients in diets rich in animal fats and the possible carcinogenic effects of cooking meat at high temperatures.

It is clear, however, that there is a correlation between the intake of dietary fat (polyunsaturated fatty acids in particular) and the incidence of prostate cancer and associated mortality. In addition, it has been demonstrated in the laboratory that a diet low in animal fat can reduce the growth of cancer cells and, conversely, that high levels of dietary fat can stimulate growth of prostate cancer cells.

Calcium surplus and vitamin D deficiency

Vitamin D promotes the body's absorption of calcium, which is essential for the normal development and maintenance of bones and teeth. The body must maintain an adequate level of calcium in order to form and sustain strong bones, especially in children and the elderly.

There are two sources of vitamin D: food (mainly eggs, butter, liver and fatty fish) and synthesis by the body in the skin on exposure to ultraviolet rays from the sun. Sunlight stimulates the body to produce vitamin D. Vitamin D is unusual in that, unlike other vitamins, it is produced by the body as well as being available in food.

WHAT ARE FREE RADICALS?

The human body needs oxygen to live. Much the way cars consume gasoline and emit pollution into the environment, our cells produce energy from oxygen and nutrients, leaving behind waste products known as free radicals. And just like pollution, free radicals are toxic. As a defence, the body contains agents called anti-oxidants that effectively neutralize free radicals. They are discussed in more detail in Chapter 7.

However, some free radicals are unaffected by anti-oxidants and can therefore attack the body's cells and tissues, accelerating their aging process or even their destruction. Research has shown that free radicals are involved in the development of a number of diseases, including prostate cancer. Diets rich in animal fat are suspected of causing excess production of free radicals in the body.

There is growing evidence that vitamin D deficiency may play a role in prostate cancer development. Data suggesting a link between vitamin D deficiency and increased risk of prostate cancer can be outlined as follows:

- The Japanese have one of the lowest rates of prostate cancer, and their diet is rich in vitamin D (fish).

VITAMIN D SUPPLEMENT

Canadian Cancer Society recommendation
In 2007, the Canadian Cancer Society recommended an increase in vitamin D intake to reduce the risks of developing cancer.

Because of our northern latitude, the sun's rays are weaker in the fall and winter. We therefore recommend that Canadian adults consider taking a vitamin D supplement. Talk to your doctor about taking 1000 international units (IU) a day during fall and winter months.

It is important to understand that vitamin D supplements should be used with caution and we recommend following the Health Canada guidelines.

Who's at higher risk?
You're probably not getting enough vitamin D if you

- are over 50
- have dark skin
- don't go outside very much
- wear clothing covering most of your skin

If you fall into one of these categories, talk to your doctor about whether you should take a vitamin D supplement of 1000 IU every day, all year round.

- Consumption of dairy products that are rich in calcium have been associated with an increased risk of prostate cancer; calcium depresses blood levels of vitamin D.
- As we age, our bodies are less able to manufacture vitamin D. This may partially explain why prostate cancer develops in older men.
- African Americans have the highest rates of prostate cancer in the world. The melatonin in black skin may interfere with the synthesis of vitamin D.
- Men who live in colder countries, where there are fewer hours of sunlight, are more likely to develop prostate cancer.

CHRONIC INFLAMMATION AND INFECTION

Chronic inflammation and infection play a role in many cancers, and there is a growing body of evidence which suggests a similar process may be involved in prostate cancer. Studies have shown a higher prostate cancer risk in men with a history of sexually transmitted disease or prostatitis.

Infections and chronic inflammation lead to repeated prostate tissue damage and repair. It is believed that the body may release free radicals during the repair process. In turn, these free radicals are believed to increase cancer development. Genetic susceptibility to chronic inflammation and tissue damage may also play a role.

A number of studies have concluded that anti-oxidants (substances that fight free radicals) may protect against prostate cancer (this is addressed in Chapter 7).

MALE HORMONES

Male hormones (also called androgens) influence the development and maintenance of the prostate throughout life, and they play a major role in prostate health. As noted in Chapter 1, testosterone triggers the growth of the prostate during puberty.

Prostates that are not exposed to male hormones do not develop cancer. Also, research has established that blocking testosterone causes prostate tumour regression in men with prostate cancer. It is clear, therefore, that male hormones are involved in prostate cancer. Unfortunately, there is no clear link between male hormone blood levels and prostate cancer.

A few years ago, it was believed that high blood levels of testosterone could very well be an important factor in prostate cancer development. Significantly, certain studies have shown that African-American men, who have the highest prostate cancer rate in the world, have 15 percent more testosterone than Caucasian men. Other studies, however, have shown that men with higher androgen blood levels may have a lower risk of aggressive prostate cancer.

This area of research is very active at the moment. Ideally, researchers would like to be able to analyze testosterone and

NOBEL PRIZE FOR MALE HORMONE RESEARCH

In the early 1940s, Dr. Charles Brenton Huggins, an American surgeon born in Canada, hypothesized that male hormones were largely responsible for the development and progression of prostate cancer. He recommended castration (removing the testicles) to stop testosterone production and halt the progression of the disease. Studies he carried out on dogs supported his hypothesis, and he received wide recognition from researchers in the field. The potential of Dr. Huggins' discovery resulted in his being awarded the Nobel Prize for Medicine in 1966. Thanks to medical progress, it is no longer necessary to perform castration to stop the body from producing testosterone. Other methods are discussed in detail in Chapter 5.

other male hormone levels in the prostate itself. Since it is very difficult to retrieve samples from the gland due to its location, researchers are evaluating blood hormone levels instead, on the assumption that these levels accurately reflect what is happening in the prostate tissue. The role of testosterone and other male hormones should become clearer over the next few years.

KEY POINTS TO REMEMBER

- There is no single cause of prostate cancer.
- Both genetics and the environment play a role in the development of prostate cancer.
- Most cancers are the result of many risk factors.
- Men with no risk factors can develop prostate cancer.
- The following table lists the factors known to be associated with prostate cancer and those known to be unassociated.

Known risk factors	Possible risk factors	Risk factors under study	Unassociated factors
Age Family history A diet high in red meat	A diet high in fat and dairy products A diet high in processed meats Being overweight or obese Inherited gene mutations Inflammation of the prostate Exposure to high levels of testosterone Tall adult height Exposure to pesticides Occupational exposures	Testosterone therapy Sexually transmitted infections (STIs) Lack of physical activity, sedentary behaviour Vasectomy Low levels of some dietary nutrients, including vitamin D, vitamin E and selenium	Benign prostatic hyperplasia Frequency of sexual activity Alcohol

- The Canadian Cancer Encyclopedia (see www.cancer.ca), compiled by the Canadian Cancer Society, is an excellent source for up-to-date information about cancer risks.

CHAPTER 3
DIAGNOSIS

Prostate cancer often develops without symptoms, and sufferers are frequently completely unaware they have the disease until it is detected by a doctor. (Note that this chapter discusses clinically significant cancers that are eventually diagnosed, not latent cancers that remain undetected.)

In fact, 80 percent of prostate cancers are discovered during routine medical checkups. Furthermore, those affected may feel perfectly healthy and be symptom-free regardless of the stage of the disease when detected. In some cases, the cancer even spreads to the pelvic lymph nodes or the bones without causing a single symptom. This can occur if the tumour in the prostate remains relatively small and the metastatic tumours do not become large enough to cause noticeable health problems.

Today, doctors are able to detect prostate cancer even before there is any reason to suspect its presence, thanks in large part to the prostate specific antigen (PSA) test, a screening method developed about 30 years ago (this is discussed in more detail later on in this chapter). If treatment begins early, there is a better chance of curing the disease.

Each case is evaluated according to individual factors, such as the patient's age and life expectancy based on personal and family history. These elements guide the doctor as he or she performs the initial medical work-up and determines the treatment.

SYMPTOMS OF PROSTATE CANCER

In its early stages, the disease is generally asymptomatic (presents no symptoms). In some cases, the tumour in the prostate grows and presses on the urethra, making it difficult to urinate. This can cause the following lower urinary tract symptoms (LUTS or prostatism):

- Difficulty starting the urine flow (hesitancy)
- Difficulty stopping the urine flow (dribbling)
- Decrease in the size and force of the urinary stream (weak or interrupted flow)
- Sensation that the bladder has not fully emptied
- Urgent need to urinate
- Frequent urination during the day and night

The tumour causes only urinary symptoms; no pain is felt in the prostate gland itself. It should be remembered that the symptoms listed above are generally not indicative of cancer but rather the result of the benign enlargement of the gland (benign prostatic hyperplasia), a frequent part of aging. They could also be caused by other urinary tract problems. The best way to ease your mind is to consult a doctor.

After the cancer begins to grow in the prostate, it spreads to the pelvic lymph nodes. (These are not the lymph nodes in the groin, which are perceptible to the touch. The pelvic lymph nodes are located deep in the abdomen next to the prostate and cannot be seen or felt.) This is known as nodal metastasis. Nodal metastasis is not painful, although it sometimes causes edema (swelling) of the feet and ankles due to blocked circulation in the lymphatic system, a network of vessels that run along the veins and arteries transporting lymphatic fluid to fight infections.

In more advanced stages of the disease, the cancerous cells usually migrate to the bones, particularly those of the pelvis and spinal column. This is known as bone metastasis. If extensive, the following symptoms may appear:

- Lower back or hip pain

PROSTATE CANCER SCREENING RECOMMENDATIONS

The Canadian Cancer Society recommends that every man over the age of 50 talk to his doctor about the benefits and risks of PSA and digital rectal exam (DRE) screening. The Association also recommends that men in high-risk groups (including African-Canadian men and men with a family history of prostate cancer) consult a doctor about whether to begin this testing before the age of 50.

The Prostate Cancer Canada Network advises all men over the age of 45 to insist that their doctor check for signs of prostate cancer during annual checkups. The Network also recommends that those at high risk for developing prostate cancer—for instance, men of African descent or with a family history of prostate cancer—should start being tested annually at age 40.

The Canadian Urological Association maintains that DRE and PSA testing increase the early detection of clinically significant prostate cancer, and that men should be made aware of the potential benefits and risks of early detection so they can make an informed decision about whether to be screened. The Association also maintains that prostate cancer screening should be offered to all men 50 years of age or older with at least a 10-year life expectancy.

Any man who is concerned about prostate cancer screening should discuss the subject with his doctor.

- Numbness or paralysis of the lower limbs (if the metastasis involves the spinal column, it can pinch the spinal cord)
- Edema (swelling) of the feet and ankles (nodal metastasis can lead to poor lymph drainage in the lower limbs)
- Loss of weight and general malaise (the patient does not feel well)
- Constant fatigue and pallor (bone metastasis can cause anemia)

In its final stages, the cancer metastasizes to other organs in the body and becomes generalized. Current diagnostic tests usually detect the disease before it progresses this far.

SIGNS OF PROSTATE CANCER AND THE PHYSICAL EXAMINATION

Signs are not the same as symptoms. While symptoms are experienced by the patient, signs are the objective manifestations of the disease observed by the doctor.

The digital rectal exam (DRE) is the most common and simple prostate cancer screening method. Although not painful, it is a little uncomfortable, as it involves the doctor inserting a gloved finger into the patient's rectum and palpating the gland. Since most tumours develop on the outside of the prostate, near the rectum, it is generally quite easy to detect an abnormality.

In its normal state, the prostate is smooth and rubbery. The doctor therefore checks for a lump or induration (hardening), though hardening can also be caused by other diseases (such as inflammation or benign prostatic hyperplasia) or by a calcification or "stone" in the prostate. Prostate indurations are found to be cancerous in only one in three cases. In some patients with prostate cancer, hardening is extensive and the lump can extend out beyond the prostate to neighbouring organs. These signs help the doctor to determine the stage of the disease and the appropriate treatment for the patient.

An enlarged prostate is not considered a sign of prostate cancer, because the gland commonly increases in size with age.

Although useful, the DRE is by no means a perfect diagnostic test since it does not allow the doctor to examine the entire prostate. In fact, most cases of prostate cancer diagnosed in Canada are not detected through a physical examination. Nevertheless, it is an important basic exam because it allows the doctor to evaluate the condition of the prostate and sometimes helps identify cancers that are not detected by the PSA test.

PROSTATE SPECIFIC ANTIGEN (PSA) AND THE PSA TEST

To complete the evaluation and rule out cancer, the doctor will request a blood test to measure prostate specific antigen (PSA) levels.

PSA is a glycoprotein (a protein mixed with a molecule of sugar) produced by normal prostate cells. It is generally believed that PSA helps liquefy the substances that compose semen and that this plays a role in fertility, but the role of PSA is still being researched. A certain amount of PSA is also found in the bloodstream.

The levels of this antigen vary according to age and race. The more cells there are in the prostate, the more PSA is produced. PSA levels are therefore naturally higher in men over the age of 40 because of the increased size of the gland, even if there is no cancer. In cases of cancer, PSA levels are even higher.

Normal PSA level for a Caucasian man in his sixties is between 0 and 4 nanograms per millilitre (ng/mL). If a patient's PSA level is higher than 4.0 ng/mL, there could be a problem: if it is between 4.0 ng/mL and 10.0 ng/mL and the prostate seems normal, the probability of prostate cancer is approximately 30 percent; if it is above 10.0 ng/mL, the risk of cancer is 50 percent; and if it is over 10.0 ng/mL and there is a lump on the prostate, the probability of prostate cancer increases to 80 percent.

Prostate cancer frequently causes an increase in PSA levels. When cells are normal, more of the antigen stays in the prostate and blood PSA levels remain low. Cancerous cells, on the other hand, are more disorganized and allow more PSA to leak into the bloodstream.

Doctors therefore use blood tests to measure blood PSA levels. Most patients with a tumour the size of a sugar cube (1 cm^3) or larger will have an abnormal PSA level.

It should be remembered that elevated PSA levels indicate a prostate condition but not necessarily prostate cancer. An elevated PSA level when no cancer is actually present is called a "false positive" result. In addition to age and benign prostatic hyperplasia, the possible causes of high PSA levels include inflammation of the prostate (sometimes caused by procedures that irritate the prostate, such as cystoscopy or placement of a catheter to empty the bladder) and urinary tract infection. In most cases, levels return to normal once the inflammation or infection resolves. Since cancer is only one of many possible causes for an

AGE- AND RACE-SPECIFIC UPPER LIMITS OF NORMAL FOR PSA (in nanograms per millilitre, ng/mL)

Age (years)	White	Black	Asian
40-49	2.5	2.0	2.0
50-59	3.5	4.0	3.0
60-69	4.5	4.5	4.0
70-80	6.5	5.5	5.0

Remember that these are approximate values and that there is no need to jump to conclusions if your PSA values differ. Always discuss your results with your doctor.

Source: Wein AJ et al., *Campbell-Walsh Urology*, 9th edition (St. Louis: W.B Saunders, 2007)

increase in PSA, it is important not to jump to conclusions. It should be noted, however, that a DRE very rarely causes PSA elevation.

This said, PSA levels can also be normal in patients who have prostate cancer. According to a study published in 2004 in the New England Journal of Medicine, PSA levels remain normal in 15 percent of men who have the disease. This result is known as a "false negative."

The PSA test is the best screening method available—it increases early detection of anomalies, and is simple, quick and more accurate than many tests available for other types of cancer. Nevertheless, it is not perfect. There has therefore been a significant amount of research done to refine the measurement of PSA in the blood, increase the accuracy of the test and reduce the number of false negative and false positive results. The following four methods have been developed:

- **PSA density measurement**. The first step in determining PSA density involves using a transrectal ultrasound to measure prostate size. Expected PSA levels are then calculated according to the size of the gland (the larger the gland, the higher the level) and compared to the patient's actual PSA level. There is an increased probability of prostate cancer if PSA density is higher than predicted.
- **Free PSA testing and total PSA testing**. A variant of the PSA test measures only "free" PSA—in other words, PSA which circulates freely in the blood and is not bound to other proteins. A total, or inclusive, test measures both types. It is believed that the more specific blood analysis of a free PSA test may help prevent the false positives that sometimes result from total PSA tests. For example, it has been observed that free PSA levels are higher in men with benign prostatic hyperplasia and lower in those with prostate cancer. In these cases then, a free PSA test can eliminate the need for further testing.

- **PSA velocity testing**. Velocity refers to the speed at which PSA levels increase over time. This test involves measuring PSA blood levels over several months or years, since an unexpected increase is sometimes the only indication of prostate cancer. For example, a PSA level that spikes suddenly from 1.0 to 3.0 is suspicious, while a level that remains constant at 3.0 is considered normal. This is why a growing number of men are asking their doctors for regular PSA testing.
- **Age-specific upper limit of normal for PSA**. PSA levels vary with age and tend to increase as a man grows older. Urologists are increasingly using age-related "normal" PSA levels in interpreting PSA results. To improve detection of significant cancer, it seems that a PSA < 4.0 ng/mL should be considered normal in younger men.

TRANSRECTAL ULTRASOUND (TRUS) AND PROSTATE BIOPSY

Although the DRE and PSA tests are useful, they are not enough to make a clear diagnosis of prostate cancer. When results are abnormal or questionable, the doctor may prescribe a transrectal ultrasound and a biopsy. These tests usually provide enough information for a precise diagnosis.

Transrectal ultrasound (TRUS)

During a transrectal ultrasound, the doctor inserts an instrument fitted with a biopsy needle into the rectum. The instrument directs sound waves toward the prostate to create an image of the gland (Figure ❶). The procedure takes only a few minutes and requires no special preparation. Although not painful, it is rather uncomfortable (much like a DRE). The TRUS is not sufficiently precise to confirm the presence of a tumour, but it can

CHAPTER 3 – DIAGNOSIS 61

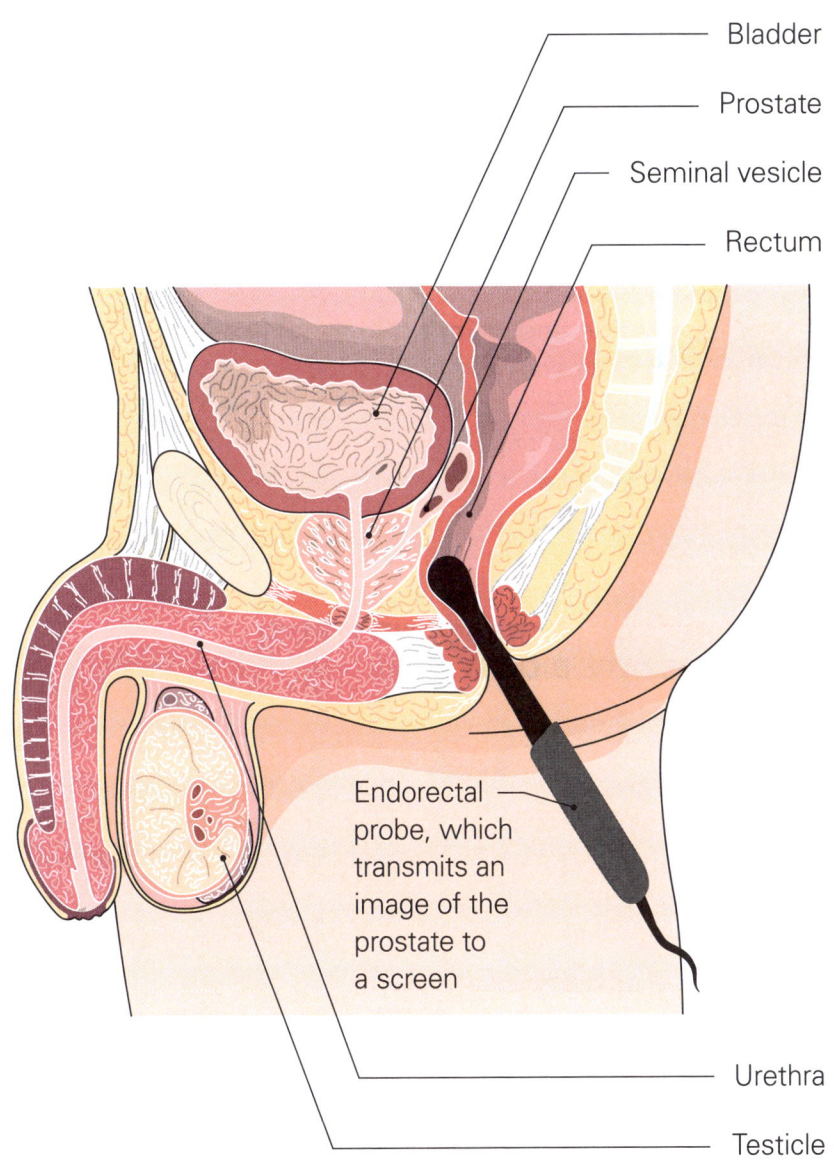

❶ Transrectal ultrasound

help the doctor measure the size of the prostate and detect any abnormalities requiring biopsy.

The TRUS is also used in biopsy procedures (TRUS-guided biopsy) to help guide the needle as it pierces the rectum wall and moves toward the different areas of the prostate where tissue samples are collected. Up until only a few years ago, doctors collected no more than six biopsy samples and frequently missed affected areas. Current practice is more effective, involving anywhere from six to twelve samples.

Prostate biopsy

Although the biopsy procedure is rather uncomfortable, it is not painful and takes only five to ten minutes. Immediately following the procedure, patients may develop lower abdominal cramps, but these generally last no more than ten minutes. In some cases, the patient will find blood in his urine, semen or stools due to the tiny rectal perforations made by the needle.

THE PATHOLOGIST

A pathologist is a medical specialist who studies human tissue. The pathologist's primary role is to make diagnoses based on a microscopic analysis of tissue samples (biopsy).

The samples of prostate or pelvic lymph node tissue removed by a urologist or radiologist for biopsy are analyzed by a pathologist to ascertain whether they are cancerous.

The pathologist also determines the grade of the tumour, an important factor in determining the aggressiveness of the cancer. This specialist's contribution is essential, as it helps the attending physician develop an effective treatment adapted to the individual patient.

This is generally harmless and disappears after a few days or weeks.

Occasionally, bacteria from the rectum travel with the needle into the gland and cause an infection in the prostate, one of the more serious possible consequences of biopsy. In these cases, the patient experiences a general malaise and develops a fever. Bacterial infections are treated with antibiotics. Such cases are infrequent, affecting from 1 to 4 percent of those who undergo prostate biopsies. Most infections are linked to bacteria that are resistant to the standard antibiotics used to prevent infection.

ADDITIONAL TESTS

If the biopsy confirms the presence of a tumour, additional tests may be required to determine whether the cancerous cells have spread elsewhere in the body. These are generally undergone by men presenting serious signs of the disease, such as an extensive induration or lump in the prostate, elevated PSA levels or biopsy results indicating the presence of an aggressive cancer.

Lymphadenectomy
A pelvic lymphadenectomy (or lymph node dissection) is a diagnostic surgical procedure performed under general anesthesia to determine whether nodal metastasis has occurred. In other words, it involves taking tissue samples from the pelvic lymph nodes to see whether the prostate cancer has spread to this area. A lymphadenectomy is usually performed at the same time as a radical prostatectomy (removal of the prostate to treat localized cancer). A pelvic lymphadenectomy alone may be performed in some cases, such as when a doctor wishes to know how far the cancer has spread before sending the patient to radiation therapy.

Bone scan
A bone scan is a nuclear medicine procedure involving injection of a radioactive isotope (a harmless radioactive substance) that allows the doctor to see if the cancer has spread to the bones (bone metastases). The procedure is painless and safe (Figure ❷).

CT scan
Some patients ask the doctor whether transaxial tomography, more commonly known as a CT scan or CAT scan, would be useful. This is a radiological exam that generates a precise image of the chest, abdomen and pelvic area and may be used to determine if the cancer has spread to the lymph nodes or to other organs such as the liver or the lungs. CT scans are commonly performed in colon, liver or pancreatic cancers but are only used in prostate cancer if the patient is at risk of metastasis, as determined by looking at PSA levels, Gleason score and DRE findings. When the risk is believed to be low, doctors will not routinely order CT scans to screen for metastasis.

CT scans are, nonetheless, often used by radiation oncologists who need to know the exact size and shape of the prostate to guide radiation therapy for prostate cancer. However, these scans are not usually precise enough to help in visualizing the cancer within the prostate or in evaluating the extent (stage) of the disease. A better option for evaluating the prostate itself is the mpMRI (see below).

Multiparametric magnetic resonance imaging (mpMRI)
Multiparametric magnetic resonance imaging (mpMRI) is a sophisticated radiological imaging technique that uses magnetic forces, radiofrequency waves and a computer to make detailed 3D images of the prostate and its surroundings. The hope is that this imaging technique will enable more precise biopsy of

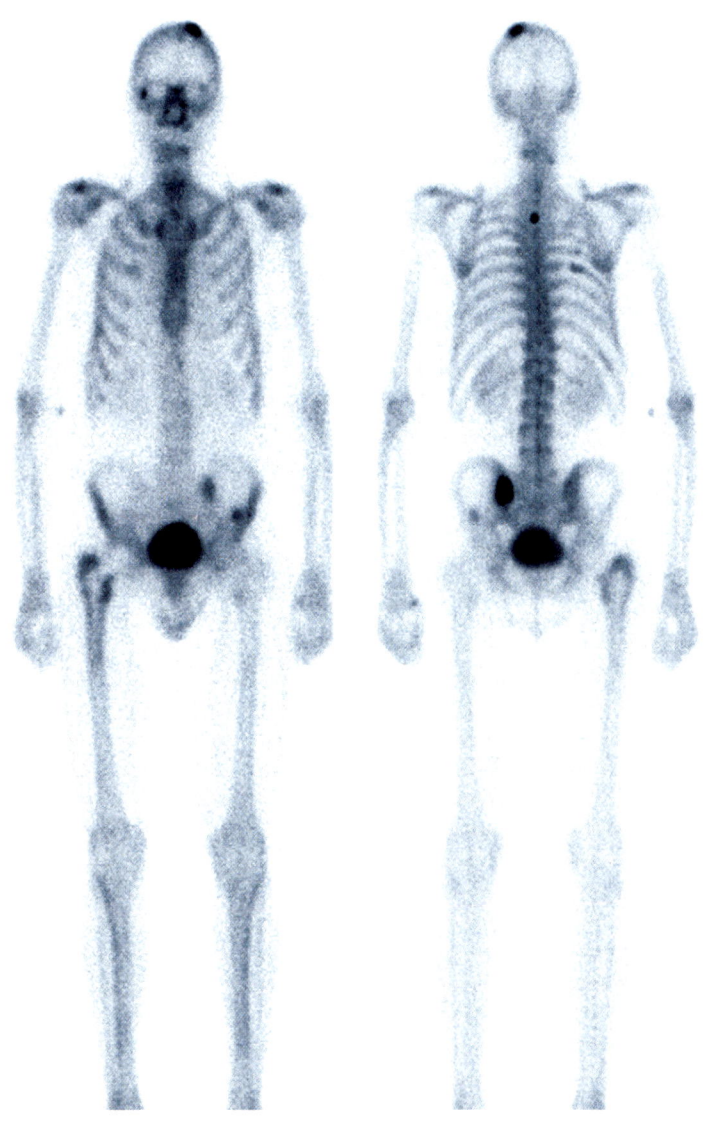

❷ Bone scan

areas with cancer and minimize unnecessary biopsies in patients without life-threatening cancer. Researchers are currently studying when to use a prostate mpMRI in clinical practice. In 2017, the Canadian Urological Association (CUA) recommended that patients with a prior negative TRUS-guided biopsy (see "Transrectal ultrasound" above) who demonstrate increasing risk of clinically significant prostate cancer may benefit from an mpMRI prior to repeat biopsy.

The Canadian Cancer Society says an mpMRI can be used to:

- Look for cancer in the front of the prostate that may be missed with other tests
- Look for prostate cancer when the doctor thinks it might be present but it isn't found with a biopsy
- Measure the size of the prostate or a tumour in the prostate
- Plan radiation therapy to treat prostate cancer
- Guide the needle during a prostate biopsy
- See if cancer has spread outside of the prostate

When to use an mpMRI is still under study, and its use in managing prostate cancer is evolving. There is no doubt that this imaging technique will be increasingly useful in managing prostate cancer in the future.

Fusion biopsies

In recent years, prostate biopsies have been performed by "fusing" mpMRI images with live, real-time ultrasound images of the prostate. A patient first has an mpMRI. The image obtained is then superimposed or "fused" with a real-time ultrasound image of the prostate to guide the biopsy. It is hoped that fusion biopsies will improve our ability to detect prostate cancer when present, reducing the risks of false negative results (that is, missing a cancer when there is one present).

Prostate-specific membrane antigen positron emission tomography (PSMA-PET)

Positron emission tomography (PET) is a medical imaging technique that is widely used to diagnose cancers. Before the scan, a radioactive material (18F-FDG) is injected into the patient's body to make it possible to specifically target and visualize cancerous cells from the radioactive emissions of this material. Most cancerous cells absorb glucose, and since 18F-FDG is similar to glucose, the cancerous cells will absorb it and can then be detected. PET scans are not, however, very helpful in prostate cancer, because prostate cancer cells absorb very little glucose.

PSMA-PET, or prostate-specific membrane antigen positron emission tomography, is a recent innovation that specifically seeks out cancerous cells of prostatic origin. A protein (prostate specific membrane antigen, or PSMA), is normally expressed on the surface of the cells of the prostate. However, PSMA expression is much higher in cancerous prostate cells than in normal prostate cells. PSMA-PET uses a radioactive material that targets PSMA rather than glucose, the target of a conventional PET scan, and can thus specifically pinpoint cancerous cells of prostatic origin. This means the doctor can get a more accurate picture of the spread of the disease throughout the patient's body (Figure ❸). Studies are currently in progress to determine if PSMA-PET will mean changing the treatment suggested for certain patients.

Note, however, that this test is still in the experimental phase and is not routine in the management of prostate cancer.

CLASSIFICATION OF PROSTATE CANCER

Prostate cancer treatment depends in large part on the degree to which the cancer cells have propagated. It is therefore useful to determine the grade and stage of the cancer and hence the risk of metastasis and eventual progression.

Grading and staging indicate the degree to which the disease has progressed at the time of diagnosis. For example, the cancerous cells may be aggressive (score 8) but still confined to the prostate (stage T2), or conversely, they may appear almost normal (score 6) but have already spread to the bones (stage M1). Every case of prostate cancer is different, and it is difficult to predict how the disease will progress.

PSA level and cancer grade and stage are key factors taken into account when treatment options are presented to the patient. However, doctors must also consider the patient's age, general health, medical history and personal preferences before deciding on treatment.

Grading

"Grade" refers to the malignancy (or aggressiveness) of the cancer based on the appearance of the prostate tissue. Grade is scored from one to five on the Gleason scale, developed in 1966 by Dr. Donald F. Gleason, a pathologist from the University of Minnesota, to evaluate cancerous cells. The Gleason scale is used for all types of cancer.

If the tissue is still very similar in appearance to that of a healthy gland, the pathologist classifies the cancer as grade 1 or 2. If the tissue has a significantly irregular appearance, it is given a grade of 4 or 5. Grade 3 is considered intermediate.

Specifically, the pathologist uses a microscope to examine biopsy samples and assigns two grades to the tissue. This is necessary because prostate tissue is rarely homogeneous throughout the gland and there may be areas where the cancer is more aggressive, even within the same tissue sample. Assigning two grades, therefore, provides a more accurate picture of the disease. The first grade is the primary or most common grade in the sample, and the second is the secondary or second most common grade. The two are added together, and the total is known as the "score."

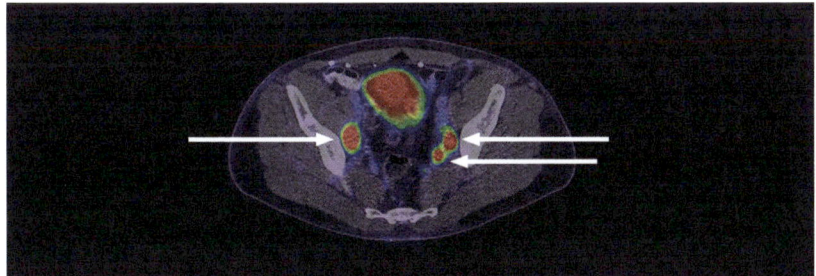
Three pelvic lymph node metastases

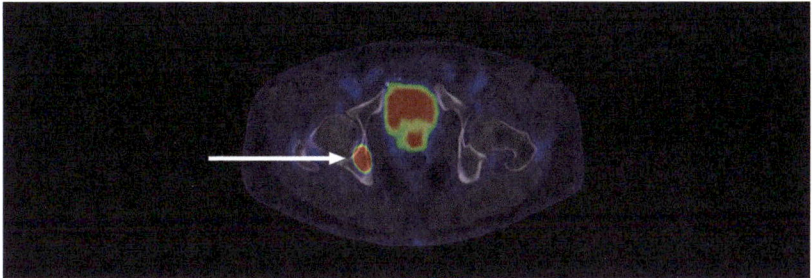
Single bone metastasis in the pelvic region

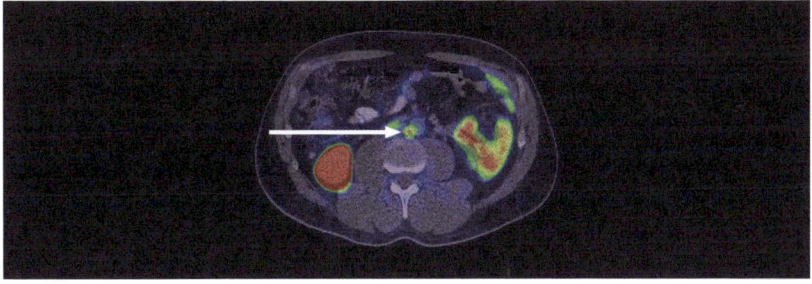
Metastasis in a tiny (2-mm) node in the abdomen undetectable by other investigations

❸ Prostate-specific membrane antigen positron emission tomography (PSMA-PET)

The order of the individual numbers is also important. For example, the patient whose total score is 7 with individual grades of 3 + 4 has a less aggressive cancer than another with a score of 7 and individual grades of 4 + 3. This makes a difference when choosing the appropriate treatment and predicting the risk of recurrence following treatment.

If the tissue sample is the same grade throughout, the score is simply double the grade (3 + 3, for example, for a score of 6). It should also be noted that the more aggressive the cancer, the less likely it is that there will be a significant variation of grades within any one sample. It is therefore practically impossible to receive a score of 5 + 1 or even 4 + 2.

Generally, high grades and scores correspond to rapidly growing tumours and indicate a poorer prognosis.

Staging

The "stage" of the cancer (Figure ❹) refers to the degree to which the cancer has spread. In the early stages, the cancer is confined within the gland. In the intermediate stages, the local tumour begins to extend beyond the prostate. In advanced and very advanced stages, the cancerous cells invade other tissues, notably the pelvic nodes and the bones. In other words, the cancer metastasizes. Later, the cancer becomes generalized throughout the entire body.

The most commonly used system to classify the stages of prostate cancer is the international TNM (Tumour, Node, Metastasis) system. "T" refers to the size of the tumour in the prostate itself, "N" describes the degree of lymph node involvement, and "M" refers to the presence or absence of metastases far from the tumour. There are other staging systems, but this is the one preferred by the Canadian medical community.

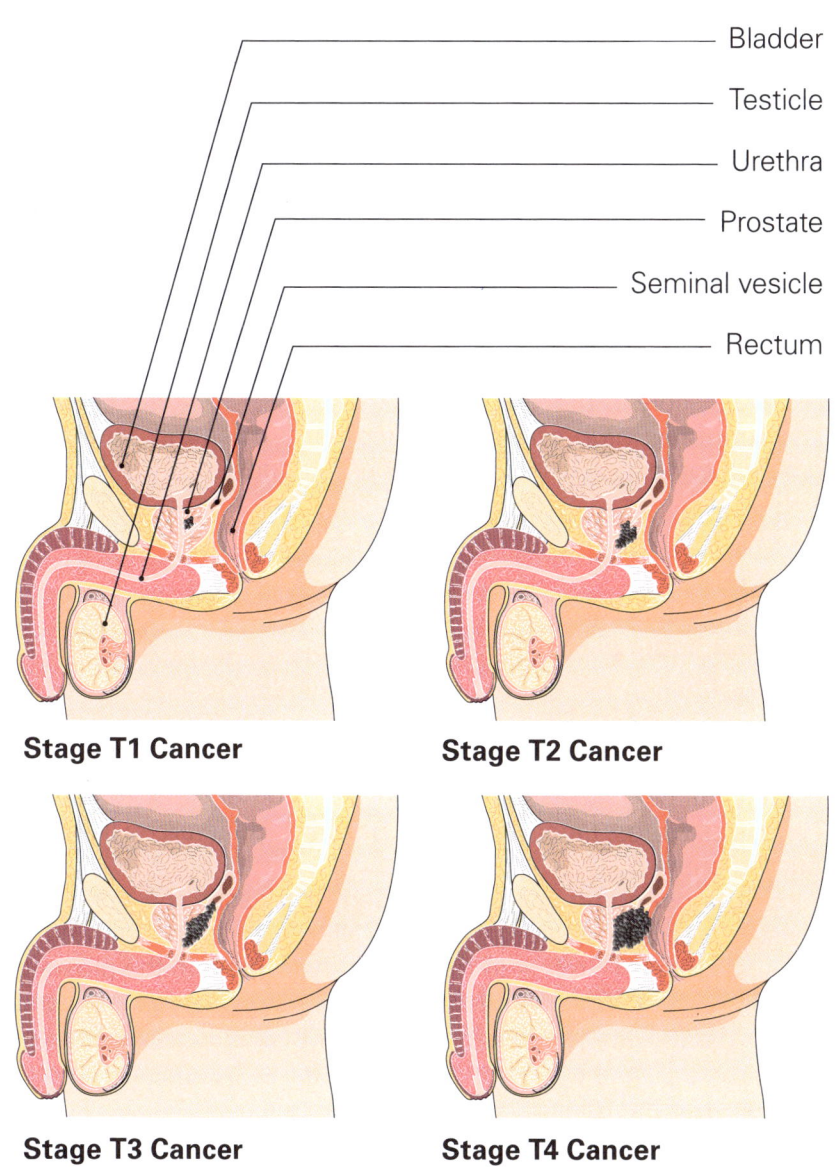

❹ Different stages of prostate cancer

GRADING AND STAGING OF PROSTATE CANCER

Gleason grades

Grade 1: The tissue is still quite similar in appearance to healthy tissue; this is the least aggressive grade.
Grade 2: The tissue is a little different from normal tissue.
Grade 3: The tissue is moderately different from normal tissue.
Grade 4: The tissue is abnormally shaped and quite irregular.
Grade 5: The tissue is very different from normal tissue; this is the most aggressive grade.

Because prostate gland tissue is rarely homogeneous, the cancer may be more aggressive in some areas than others. Doctors therefore calculate two individual grades to get a more complete picture of the disease. The total of the two grades is known as the score.

TNM stages

T (size of the tumour in the prostate)
T0 There is no evidence of tumour in the prostate.
T1 The prostate seems normal and the tumour was discovered due to a high PSA measurement.
T2 The tumour is palpable and confined within the prostate.
T3 The tumour extends beyond the prostate (affecting the capsule, that is, the tissue surrounding the gland, and/or the seminal vesicles).
T4 The tumour has invaded neighbouring tissues (bladder neck, external sphincter, rectum, etc.).

N (degree of lymph node involvement)
N0 There is no evidence of a tumour in the lymph nodes.
N+ One or more lymph nodes are involved.

M (presence or absence of further metastases)
M0 There is no metastasis beyond the lymph nodes.
M1 There is bone or distant metastasis.

KEY POINTS TO REMEMBER

- Eighty percent of prostate cancer cases are discovered during a routine examination that includes a PSA test. Whether the disease is in its early or advanced stages when detected, the patient may still feel perfectly healthy and be symptom-free.

- Lower urinary tract symptoms (LUTS or prostatism) do not necessarily indicate prostate cancer. They can also be caused by other urinary tract problems.

- Although useful, the DRE is not a perfect diagnostic test since the doctor cannot examine the entire prostate using this method. Most cases of prostate cancer diagnosed in Canada are not detected through a physical examination. However, a DRE can sometimes "catch" cases that would not have been detected by a PSA test.

- Thanks to the PSA test, doctors can detect prostate cancer before there is any reason to suspect its presence. As a result, treatment can begin earlier and patients stand a better chance of being cured.

- For every three tests showing abnormally high PSA levels, only one is caused by prostate cancer. Fifteen percent of men with prostate cancer have normal PSA levels.

- Biopsy usually leads to an accurate diagnosis.

- The choice of treatment depends on the patient's age, general state of health, medical history and personal preferences.

TWO PEOPLE'S STORIES

Name: Frank   **Age:** 63 years old

Occupation: Retired accountant

Frank is retired and in good health. He keeps busy with leisure activities, sports, volunteer work and his grandchildren. He has always been concerned with good nutrition and watches what he eats.

During a routine examination, his doctor detected a lump extending beyond the prostate and found his PSA level to be 23.0 ng/mL, five times higher than normal. A TRUS revealed a suspicious abnormality that appeared to extend beyond the capsule (envelope surrounding the prostate). Several biopsies were done in this area, and the pathologist determined that Frank has a grade 4+5 (score of 9) cancer. Frank had a CT scan that revealed the cancer had spread to the lymph nodes in his pelvis (close to the prostate). A biopsy confirmed the presence of cancer in the lymph nodes. The bone scan was normal.

What's going on? Frank has fairly advanced prostate cancer that has spread to the pelvic lymph nodes (N1) but not yet to the bones (M0). It is now up to him and his doctor to choose the appropriate treatment, which may include hormone therapy and possibly radiation therapy. The chance of cure is low, but given all the options to treat his cancer, Frank is likely to live many years with a very good quality of life. It is important to remain optimistic even if cure is not always possible. Progress is being made in changing prostate cancer from a life-threatening disease to a chronic and controllable disease.

CHAPTER 3 – DIAGNOSIS

Name: Charles	**Age:** 50 years old
Occupation: Businessman	

Charles works 40 hours a week, plays golf and jogs. During his last annual check-up, his doctor performed a digital rectal exam (DRE), and everything seemed normal. However, his PSA test results were a little high at 5.0 ng/mL.

The doctor carried out a transrectal ultrasound (TRUS), found no abnormalities and collected some samples for biopsy. The pathologist determined that the prostate contained cancerous cells scoring 7 (grades 3 + 4) on the Gleason scale. Additional tests came up negative.

What does it all mean? While the DRE and the TRUS showed nothing, Charles does have cancer, although it is not very advanced. His options included radiation therapy and radical prostatectomy. Charles opted for surgery and the pathological tissue analysis showed his cancer was confined to the prostate (T2) and had not spread to the pelvic lymph nodes (N0).

Charles has an excellent chance of being cured and will likely not require other treatment.

CHAPTER 4
TREATMENT OF LOCALIZED PROSTATE CANCER

Prostate cancer is said to be localized when the cancer does not appear to have spread outside the gland and affects no other organ (no metastases). Treating this type of cancer is a complex task because so many factors need to be taken into account.

The first issue to consider is the grade, which indicates the aggressiveness of the tumour and is determined by the appearance of the tissue under a microscope. The next is the stage, the extent to which the cancer has invaded the prostate, which is assessed through a digital rectal exam (DRE). Another crucial factor is the patient's prostate specific antigen (PSA) blood level, so far the most accurate indicator of the aggressiveness of prostate cancer (see boxes in Chapter 3, "Age- and race-specific upper limits of normal for PSA" and "Grading and staging of prostate Cancer").

These elements help the doctor evaluate the tumour and the risk of death from the disease in the years to come. Of course, the patient's age is also considered, along with his life expectancy and his medical and family history.

If the cancer is caught early, remains confined to the prostate and is treated in a timely manner, it can generally be cured. In some cases, however, treatment can actually do more harm than good, causing side effects and complications more distressing than the disease itself— particularly if the cancer is very slow growing. Surprising as it may seem, therefore, sometimes the best treatment is no treatment at all!

Combination therapy is often recommended if prostate cancer becomes locally advanced. The doctor identifies this type of cancer by the presence of one of the following: a score of 7 or higher on the Gleason scale (an aggressive tumour); a PSA level of 20 ng/mL or more; or a stage T3 tumour (extending beyond the prostate capsule).

SELECTING A TREATMENT

The numerous factors to consider make the decision regarding treatment one of the most difficult tasks facing the patient. A great deal of information and support will be required from the doctor, and any treatment eventually embarked upon must consider the individual patient's opinions, preferences and quality-of-life expectations.

The patient should ask as many questions as he can about the disease, his life expectancy and the available treatments. He is strongly advised to take the time to reflect carefully, weigh the pros and cons of each option, gather as much information as possible and discuss the issues with his family. If he feels the need, he should not hesitate to consult another doctor for a second opinion.

CHAPTER 4 – TREATMENT OF LOCALIZED PROSTATE CANCER

There is no ready-made solution when it comes to the treatment of localized prostate cancer. Nothing is written in stone, and the treatment will depend not only on the patient's careful deliberations, but also on the doctor's approach in trying to achieve the best results for his patient. Two men with identical tumours, therefore, will not necessarily receive the same treatment.

Doctors cannot accurately predict the risk of progression of a localized prostate cancer, although they do have some tools to help guide the patient, namely the Partin tables, the Kattan nomograms and the Albertsen life tables (see the end of this chapter). These valuable prognostic models help predict the risk to the patent presented by the disease. These tables are only used for prostate cancer and cannot be applied to other types of cancers.

However, these scales are not foolproof, and the cancer may be more extensive than suspected. In some cases, the doctor discovers during or after a radical prostatectomy that the cancer has spread beyond the capsule (tissue surrounding the prostate), that the tissue margins are positive (the cancer has reached the edges of the tissue removed), that the seminal vesicles have been affected or that the cancer is present in the lymph nodes. The cancer is, of course, then assigned a different stage accordingly.

THE PATIENT'S OPTIONS

The options for patients suffering from localized prostate cancer are active surveillance, radical prostatectomy (removal of the prostate, possibly preceded by removal of lymph nodes to determine whether the cancer has spread) and radiation therapy (external beam or brachytherapy). Watchful waiting is an option for patients who are older or have other significant health problems. If the cancer is locally advanced, the doctor may recommend combination therapy that might include radical prostatectomy, radiation therapy and hormone therapy. Hormone therapy alone cannot cure cancer and must be combined with radical prostatectomy or radiation therapy for there to be a hope of beating the disease.

It is worth repeating that treatment options depend on the grade and stage of the tumour and the patient's life expectancy, which is linked to his age and general health. For example, a man under 70 years of age generally has a longer life expectancy than an older man, and if he is in good health otherwise, he can expect to live at least another 10 years.

QUESTIONS TO ASK THE DOCTOR

- What kind of cancer do I have? Is it confined to the prostate or has it started to spread or metastasize?
- Is the tumour aggressive? What is the grade of the cancer?
- Should I have any other tests?
- What are my treatment options? What factors are you considering? What treatment do you recommend?
- What are the advantages and drawbacks of each treatment?
- Do the treatments have long-term consequences, and if so, what are they? How likely am I to suffer from these consequences? Can they be prevented or treated?
- What are the chances of curing the cancer? What do we do if it comes back?
- Do you have the necessary skills to treat it, or should I consult another expert?
- Do I have to stop working during treatment?
- Do I have to change my lifestyle during treatment? What should I change, and why?
- Can I still have a sex life during and after treatment?

Men with a life expectancy of more than 10 years (generally men under the age of 70)

Relatively young men (diagnosed in their fifties and sixties) are more likely to die from prostate cancer than older men. This is not because the disease is more aggressive, but because younger men generally do not suffer from other potentially fatal conditions. Furthermore, because they have more years ahead of them, the disease has more time to develop and spread. Doctors therefore usually suggest aggressive treatments to get rid of the disease as quickly as possible.

In most cases, radical prostatectomy or radiation therapy is quite effective for tumours that do not extend beyond the prostate. Indeed, cure rates are very high in the first five to ten years after treatment. Several studies have shown that the two treatments result in a comparable quality of life (with respect to side effects and complications) after one year. After 10 years, recurrences seem to be less common for men who opted for radical prostatectomy.

In cases of locally advanced cancer (i.e., an aggressive tumour and a high score on the Gleason scale), the doctor may suggest combination therapy when PSA levels are high or the tumour seems to extend beyond the prostate. Treatment options include radical prostatectomy, radiation therapy, hormone therapy or a combination of two or all three of these therapies. For instance, if the doctor operates and finds that the cancer does indeed extend beyond the prostate, radiation therapy or hormone therapy could be added following the radical prostatectomy to improve the patient's chances (the more the tumour extends beyond the prostate, the higher the risk of recurrence). Hopefully, this is an approach that may lead to a greater chance of curing the cancer and avoiding a recurrence.

Men who suffer from serious illnesses in addition to the cancer are often poor candidates for radical prostatectomy, since it is a fairly serious operation. Watchful waiting or active surveillance is recommended in these cases if the tumour does not appear to be aggressive. Hormone and/or radiation therapy is prescribed if the tumour seems more threatening.

Radiation therapy, on the other hand, can be given to any man, no matter what his general state of health. However, radiation limits a patient's options should the cancer reappear. Specifically, radical prostatectomy is very difficult after radiation treatment because the radiation burns the prostate and surrounding tissue, reducing them to fibrotic tissue that may be difficult to remove without serious consequences. This is an important factor to consider when choosing treatment, particularly for younger patients who have more time for the cancer to recur. It should also be remembered that undergoing these treatments in the opposite order does not cause the same complications; that is, radiation therapy can often be used to treat a recurrence after a radical prostatectomy without significant problems.

Men with a life expectancy of less than 10 years (generally men over the age of 70)

For men over the age of 70 with slow-growing localized cancer, watchful waiting or active surveillance is often the recommended treatment. Indeed, in some cases the cancer progresses so slowly that the disadvantages of treatment outweigh the benefits, causing side effects that are worse than the symptoms of the disease. In addition, the older the patient, the more likely it is that he will suffer from another fatal condition before the cancer becomes a real threat.

It is therefore often wiser to wait and let the patient live normally than to subject him to the possible side effects of treatment. In most cases, there will be time to intervene with hormone therapy if the cancer starts to progress more quickly. Hormone therapy slows down the development of the disease in the entire body and alleviates symptoms. For some patients, it is sufficient treatment on its own.

Radiation therapy is also an option if the tumour is still at an early enough stage for a cure or if the cancer can be prevented from progressing and causing symptoms or from spreading if it is more aggressive.

In some situations, even in patients over 70, the doctor may recommend radical prostatectomy. This is most likely in the case of an aggressive tumour in a patient who is still in good health and has several years of life expectancy.

If the cancer has begun to extend beyond the prostate gland or seems more aggressive and surgery is not indicated, the doctor could recommend radiation therapy, hormone therapy or both.

TWO PEOPLE'S STORIES

Name: Louis	**Age:** 64 years old

Occupation: Foreman in a paper-pulp mill

Louis' prostate cancer scores 6 (grades 3 + 3) on the Gleason scale and his PSA level is 8 ng/mL. According to the Albertsen life tables analysis, there is a 68 percent risk that he will die within the next 15 years and a 23 percent chance that this will be due to prostate cancer; therefore, his chance of dying from other causes within this period is 45 percent. In other words, Louis is twice as likely to die of a cause other than prostate cancer sometime over the next 15 years.

The doctor suggests Louis opt for active surveillance instead of immediate treatment with its possible side effects. Louis doesn't agree, however; he cannot imagine living with the sword of Damocles hanging over his head and insists on treatment. The doctor proposes surgery or radiation therapy, explaining the advantages and drawbacks of both. The doctor also uses the Kattan nomograms to calculate the risk of recurrence.

Name: Larry	**Age:** 67 years old

Occupation: Sales representative

Larry plans to retire next year, buy a sailboat and travel the South Seas with his wife. Suddenly, his doctor informs him that he has localized prostate cancer, although it does not appear to be too aggressive. The tumour is at stage T1 and scores 6 (grades 3 +3) on the Gleason scale, and his PSA level is 5. The doctor presents the three treatment options—active surveillance , radical prostatectomy and radiation therapy—explaining the benefits and drawbacks of each.

Larry is unsure. He takes his time to think about it, eventually deciding on active surveillance. Because it is likely that his cancer will progress slowly, he prefers to postpone treatment and enjoy his long-anticipated trip. He will see his doctor as soon as he gets back.

WATCHFUL WAITING AND ACTIVE SURVEILLANCE

In some cases, the doctor will discover a cancer that is confined to the prostate but will recommend waiting before beginning treatment. This may seem strange, but there is a perfectly good explanation.

Prostate cancer often progresses very slowly. It can be present for years and never spread, produce symptoms or threaten the life of the patient.

Watchful waiting

Older men or men with a slow-growing cancer who have other major health problems may very likely die of another condition before the cancer becomes a threat. When all signs indicate the cancer is slow growing, the selected course of action may be to wait for symptoms to appear before beginning treatment. This is called watchful waiting. It is important in certain cases to weigh the inconvenience of treatment with the risk posed by the cancer.

Active surveillance

Active surveillance may be offered to healthy men of all ages with early stage, low-grade cancers that are likely to be slow growing. This way, the risks of erectile dysfunction and incontinence due to treatment can be avoided (at least temporarily).

Active surveillance involves regular monitoring (every three to six months) to follow the progression of the disease: digital rectal examinations (DRE), blood tests to measure PSA levels and repeated prostate biopsies are performed. Since different areas of the prostate are biopsied, disease progression can be estimated by the number of biopsies that contain cancer and whether the grade has increased in certain areas. If the cancer appears to be growing more rapidly or, more importantly, if there are changes in the grade, the doctor will recommend active treatment (radical prostatectomy or radiation and/or hormone therapy). About 25 to 50 percent of men under active surveillance are eventually treated because there are signs of cancer progression.

Although active surveillance is not really a treatment in itself, it can still present risks. The disease may begin to progress more rapidly than expected and reach an incurable stage before the doctor has had a chance to react. This does not occur very often, but patients must be aware of the risk—and of the fact that there is no 100-percent-reliable tool for predicting the progression of the disease.

RADICAL PROSTATECTOMY (REMOVAL OF THE PROSTATE GLAND)

Radical prostatectomy is a surgical procedure performed under general or spinal anesthesia that involves the complete removal of the prostate (Figure ❶). (Note that this is not the procedure used to treat benign prostatic hyperplasia, which requires that only the internal section of the gland be removed.) The chances of a cure are excellent if radical prostatectomy is performed during the early stages of the disease, when it is still confined to the prostate. Once the pelvic nodes are affected, it is generally too late for surgery to be curative. Surprises at the time of surgery (that is, a surgeon begins the operation only to find that the cancer is inoperable or has spread to the lymph nodes) are rare, since most urologists use tables that combine tumour grade, PSA and stage to ascertain the stage of the cancer; in some cases, investigative techniques are used as well.

Before going through with a prostatectomy in a patient with aggressive cancer, a surgeon may first perform a pelvic lymphadenectomy (remove a sample of the pelvic lymph nodes) to determine whether the cancer has spread (similar procedures are performed for other types of cancer as well, particularly breast cancer). In certain cases, removed tissue may be sent to the pathologist while the patient is still on the operating table, and the results are received within half an hour. If the cancer has indeed spread, the surgeon may decide to halt the procedure and switch treatment plans. Knowing whether the nodes are affected

CHAPTER 4 – TREATMENT OF LOCALIZED PROSTATE CANCER   87

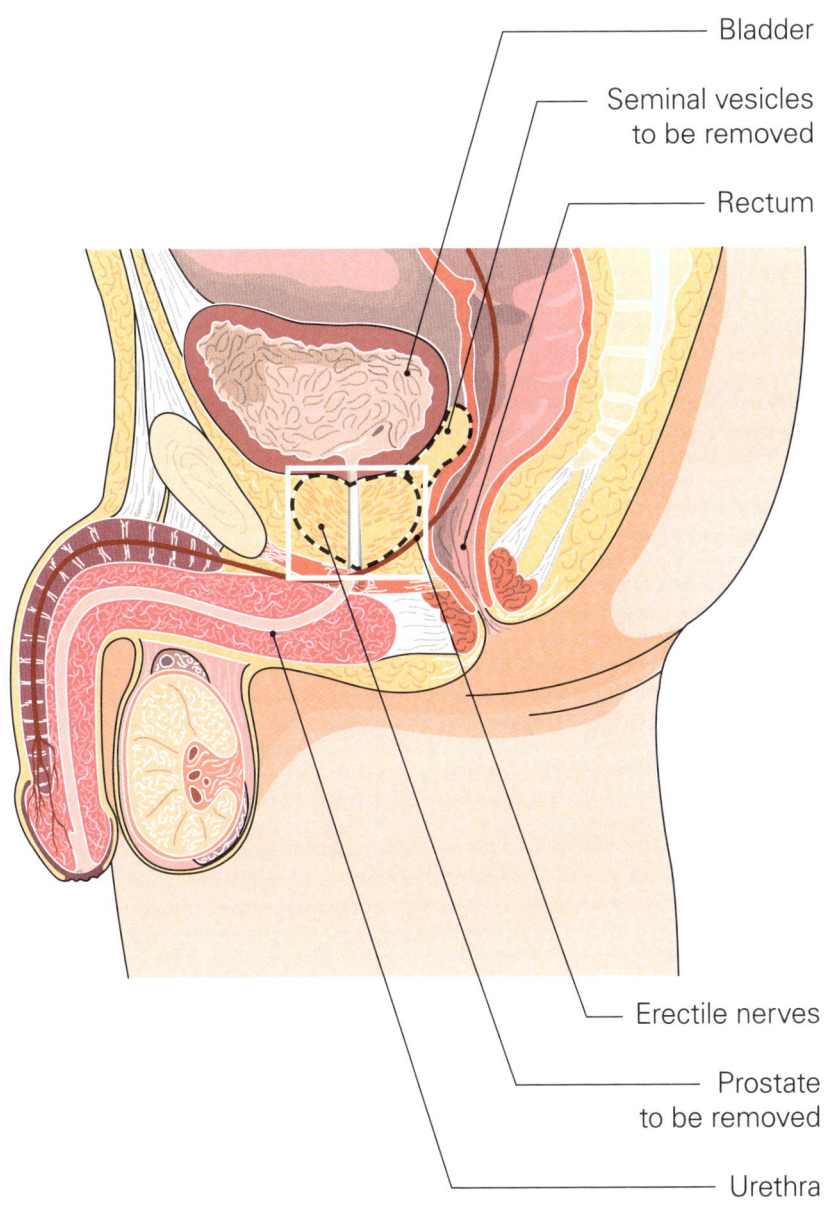

❶ Radical prostatectomy

by the cancer will influence how the patient will be followed and possibly lead to additional treatment in the short or long term.

The surgeon severs first the urethra and then the bladder neck at its junction with the prostate. The vas deferens is then cut and the prostate removed, along with some adjacent tissue. The seminal vesicles (small pouches alongside the prostate that produce substances in seminal fluid) are also removed, since cancer cells may migrate via that route. The prostate, the seminal vesicles and the tissues are then analyzed by the pathologist to determine the extent and stage of the tumour.

PRE-OPERATIVE PROCEDURES

Before surgery, the patient's general state of health must be evaluated. Doctors therefore carry out a number of tests, including blood and urine tests, an electrocardiogram (also known as an ECG) to record the electrical activity of the heart and, in some cases, radiological (X-ray) exams. These are all performed on an out-patient basis a few days or weeks before the operation.

The patient checks into the hospital the night before or the morning of the operation and may be prescribed a laxative or enema to empty his intestines. In addition, the patient must not eat or drink for eight hours before the operation.

Blood transfusions are often unnecessary, since experienced surgeons can limit the amount of blood lost during the operation. However, some hospitals ask patients to provide some of their own blood beforehand as a precautionary measure. The blood is thrown out if it is not used because hospitals do not have the right to preserve or use it for other patients. Some doctors prescribe hormone therapy prior to surgery (see the section on hormone therapy later in this chapter).

During the operation, the bladder (located right next to the prostate) is sutured directly to the urethra. The surgeon also inserts a catheter to evacuate urine while the patient heals. Care is taken to preserve the external sphincter (the muscle that surrounds the urethra and contracts to close it, controlling continence). The entire procedure takes about two hours.

In rare cases, the operation can injure the rectum, located just beside the prostate gland. This occurs in less than one percent of cases, and most of the time the surgeon corrects it immediately.

After the operation, the surgeon may insert a small tube (drain) through the abdominal wall near the incision to drain fluid from the area and prevent infection or the accumulation of fluid. In some cases, there is temporary urine leakage through the sutures joining the bladder to the urethra. Similarly, a pelvic lymphadenectomy can cause leakage of lymph from the nodes. The drain is usually left in place until there is no longer any significant drainage.

Surgical techniques

Open surgery

Traditionally, surgeons perform open radical prostatectomies through an incision in the lower abdomen (Figure ❷). Improvements to the procedure have however been made. Recent progress in surgical techniques has made it possible in some cases for experienced surgeons to identify the erectile nerves, separate them from either side of the prostate gland and thus spare them from damage during the operation. This nerve-sparing technique reduces the risk of erectile dysfunction by 50 percent (see the section below entitled "Long-term Complications of Radical Prostatectomy"), but whether or not it can be employed in any given situation depends on the size and location of the tumour; if the tumour is too large or aggressive, the nerves cannot be spared. In addition, not all surgeons use this technique, since it is more complicated and delicate than the traditional method. Patients should speak to their doctors about the procedure to be used.

Laparoscopic prostatectomy
Since the late 1990s, some treatment centres have performed laparoscopic prostatectomies. Instead of a single incision, five or six small ones (about one centimetre long) are made in the lower abdomen (Figure ❷). Long, slim surgical instruments are inserted through these incisions. A camera (endoscope) is also inserted, to guide the operation inside the abdomen. While this technique generally shortens recovery time, it is not proven to be any more effective than traditional surgery, and patients run an identical or even greater risk of incontinence and erectile problems as in open surgery. Laparoscopic prostatectomies have not gained widespread acceptance because they are technically difficult to perform even in the hands of skilled laparoscopic surgeons.

Robotic surgery
In recent years, robotic surgery has been developed and become increasingly popular. As the learning curve is faster for robotic surgery than for laparoscopy, this type of surgery is now being widely used by urological surgeons. The movements of robotic instruments are intuitive, and the surgeon has a 3D view of the prostate. In addition, robotic instruments have articulated tips which mimic human wrist movements, robotically assisted prostatectomies are minimally invasive and recovery time is shorter for patients. Unfortunately, patients still run the same risk of incontinence and erectile problems as in open surgery. There are also economic considerations with robotic surgery, and only centres with a high volume of cases can offer this technique.

Which technique is best?
Patients are thus confronted with a choice of surgical techniques. Which technique is best? The final word is not in yet.

CHAPTER 4 – TREATMENT OF LOCALIZED PROSTATE CANCER

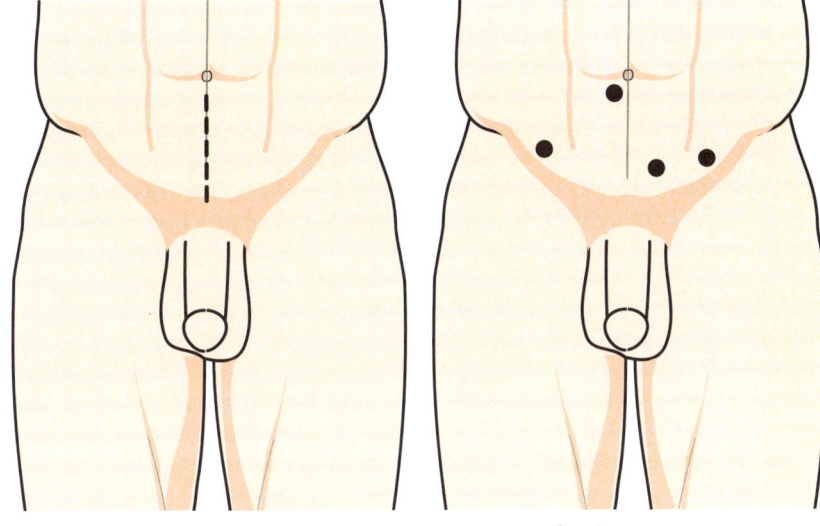

Incision for open surgery   Incisions for laparoscopy

❷ Radical prostatectomy by open surgery and laparoscopy

The most important factors are the surgeon's skill and experience, not the technique. Patients are therefore encouraged to discuss possible techniques with their doctor and to ask about his or her experience.

Short-term complications of radical prostatectomy

A radical prostatectomy operation is fairly serious and requires an average of two to five days of hospitalization and three to six weeks of convalescence at home no matter what type of surgical technique is used. There are some short-term complications.

In the first weeks after surgery, the abdominal or perineal incision will be somewhat painful. Patients who have undergone laparoscopic surgery will also experience some pain, although less pronounced. Of course, painkillers are prescribed in all cases. The patient can usually get out of bed and walk the day after the operation, resuming regular activities gradually over the next month.

After the patient is released from hospital, he wears a catheter in his urethra and a urine collection bag attached to the thigh. These are discrete and easily concealed under clothing, but they can cause some physical discomfort. In some cases, the catheter irritates the bladder wall and causes contractions, resulting in a frequent urge to urinate, even when the bladder is empty. This is a common problem that is usually not too troublesome. If necessary, your physician can prescribe medication to relax the bladder muscles.

The catheter is usually withdrawn one to two weeks after the patient returns home. Urinary incontinence is a normal short-term complication of radical prostatectomy. Most men have some trouble regaining control of the urinary mechanism and experience a frequent urge to urinate or leakage when engaging in strenuous physical activity. For 90 percent of men, things generally return to normal between one and twelve months after the operation (the average is three to six months). The patient can speed up the process by doing Kegel exercises (see "Reducing the Risk of Complications of Radical Prostatectomy" below).

Finally, radical prostatectomy, much like any other surgical operation, can lead to general complications, such as constipation caused by painkillers, pneumonia resulting from lung congestion (secretions that accumulate either during or after the operation), blood clots in the legs (phlebitis) due to immobility and wound infection.

Long-term complications of radical prostatectomy

Radical prostatectomy carries a risk of long-term complications, the primary three being erectile dysfunction (impotence), urinary incontinence and stenosis (narrowing) of the urethra.

The most common complication is erectile dysfunction. This occurs when the erectile nerves, located very near the prostate gland, are severed or damaged during the operation. In some cases, the nerves can be spared, although this is not possible if the tumour is too large, too aggressive or too close to the nerves. Furthermore, even if the doctor employs the nerve-sparing technique during surgery, there is no guarantee the patient will maintain his erectile capacity.

Right after the operation, it is practically impossible for a man to get an erection. For approximately 50 percent of men whose nerves were preserved, things return more or less to normal over the year following the procedure. The other half, if not treated, will likely experience permanent erectile dysfunction, as will nearly 100 percent of those whose nerves were not spared.

There are a number of treatments that can help men regain their erectile capacity and enjoy a satisfying sex life (see Chapter 6). However, about 10 to 15 percent of men with permanent erectile dysfunction will never be able to achieve erection, even with the help of medication. The reasons for this are not fully understood but seem to involve faulty vascularization of the penile tissue caused by the patient's general state of health. Some men choose to have penile implants permanently inserted so they can at least enjoy a more or less normal sex life.

It should be noted that a man's ability to achieve orgasm is not affected by the operation, as this ability is controlled by nerves located far from the prostate gland. The man's sex drive also remains intact, unless he undergoes hormone therapy as well (see "Hormone therapy" below). However, because the vas deferens has been severed and the prostate gland and seminal vesicles have been removed, the man is no longer able to ejaculate or, consequently, to conceive children.

Following surgery, almost all patients experience temporary incontinence. About 5 to 10 percent suffer from permanent stress incontinence, which means they sometimes experience urine leakage when they cough, laugh, sneeze or engage in strenuous physical activity (such as lifting a heavy object). Kegel exercises can be helpful in these cases (see "Reducing the Risk of Complications of Radical Prostatectomy" below).

Approximately 1 to 5 percent of men who have had a radical prostatectomy experience total and permanent urinary incontinence; that is, they are incapable of controlling their urine. In general, this occurs because the urinary sphincter (the muscle that encircles the urethra and contracts to close it) is no longer able to contract as fully as it did before the operation. In some cases, an artificial sphincter can be implanted.

The artificial urinary sphincter is a hydraulic system consisting of a silicone cuff encircling the urethra and connected to a pump located in the scrotum next to the testicles. Another tube connects the pump to a balloon reservoir which contains a saline solution and is placed in the lower abdomen. The system is surgically implanted. When the system is activated, the cuff automatically inflates with fluid and closes the urethra. The urethra thus remains closed except when the patient squeezes the control pump located in the scrotum. This pulls the fluid out from the cuff and back into the balloon reservoir, causing the sphincter to deflate and urine to flow freely from the bladder into the urethra and out of the body. The patient has one or two minutes to urinate, as fluid from the balloon reservoir will automatically flow back down to the cuff around the urethra. There are other systems to reduce or stop urine leakage. Penis clamps have been developed, as well as condom catheters that are used to collect urine leakage. Incontinence pads and pants are also greatly improved. In addition, other surgical procedures that are less extensive than an artificial sphincter are under development, such as the urethral sling and urethral compression balloons.

Stenosis of the bladder neck refers to narrowing of the diameter of the opening just below the bladder and is caused by tightening due to scar tissue between the bladder and the urethra. This condition makes urination difficult (weak urinary flow and occasional incontinence) and in some cases painful. Fortunately, this is not a serious complication and can be corrected through minor surgery (dilation and/or incision in the scar tissue). Solutions to erectile dysfunction and urinary incontinence are discussed in more detail in Chapter 6.

Reducing the risk of complications of radical prostatectomy

Recovery is easier and can be more rapid for men who do not smoke, are in good physical condition and maintain a healthy weight. It is therefore a good idea to exercise regularly and get into shape before the operation (any exercise routine should be discussed with the doctor first). Walking for half an hour every day is usually enough; it can help the patient build up physical stamina and lose extra pounds, if needed.

Pubococcygeal exercises—also known as "Kegel exercises"—should be performed regularly after the operation to reduce the risk of permanent urinary incontinence. The pubococcygeus (or PC) muscles are the ones we contract to stop urine flow. The exercises involve contracting these muscles for two to five seconds at a time while breathing normally. These exercises can be done anywhere, anytime, standing, sitting or lying down. The patient should begin practicing before the operation, to learn how to do the exercises properly, and should continue doing them during the period of convalescence. However, these exercises cannot prevent incontinence altogether. There are also perineal re-education exercises—similar to Kegel exercises, but done in the presence of a physiotherapist, who may use biofeedback, electrostimulation or manual techniques (offering resistance to push against). Perineal re-education yields better short-term results than Kegel exercises but usually must be kept up over the long term if it is to remain effective.

Deep breathing and coughing regularly can help prevent pneumonia, one of the potential complications of any type of surgery. As soon as possible after the operation, the patient should begin simply taking deep breaths, holding for five seconds and then breathing out, emptying the lungs completely. Deliberately coughing can also help dislodge any accumulated secretions caused by the artificial respiration administered during the operation. Both these exercises should be done several times a day until the patient leaves the hospital.

Once the patient returns home, he is advised to eat a balanced diet to help the body recover from the anesthesia and surgery. He should also examine the incision every day to check for redness or weeping of the wound.

Results and medical follow-up of radical prostatectomy

It is impossible to accurately estimate the general success rate of radical prostatectomy as a treatment for prostate cancer. Every man reacts differently depending on the true grade of the tumour (which can be determined only after the operation), the degree to which the cancer has spread and pre-treatment PSA levels. The less severe these three factors, the better the patient's chance of a cure.

For example, a man with a PSA level of 8 and a stage T1 tumour scoring 6 (grades 3 + 3) on the Gleason scale has a 90 percent chance of a complete cure. On the other hand, if the man has a PSA level of 10 and a stage T2 tumour scoring 7 (grades 4 + 3) on the Gleason scale, the risk of recurrence is higher. Isolated cancer cells may remain in the area formerly occupied by the prostate, eventually growing and forming a new tumour (localized recurrence).

In some cases, the doctor discovers after the operation that the cancer has extended beyond the capsule (the tissue surrounding the prostate) or that the margins are positive (the cancer has extended beyond the edge of the removed prostate tissue). In these cases, the stage of the tumour is higher than what was thought prior to surgery and the possibility of recurrence is higher.

Depending on the individual patient's risk of recurrence (either localized or distant), the doctor may suggest additional treatment (such as radiation therapy and/or hormone therapy) after the prostatectomy to reduce the risk. About one month after the operation, the patient returns to the doctor for a follow-up examination. At this visit, the doctor usually prescribes medication to help the patient regain his erectile capacity (see Chapter 6). For the first four to six weeks after surgery, the patient should avoid strenuous physical activity (such as lifting heavy objects).

Regular follow-up continues every three to six months. If everything is still fine after two to three years, annual follow-up appointments are scheduled. The doctor takes a blood test to measure PSA level at every visit, since this is the most accurate indicator of recurrence and performs occasional digital rectal exams. After the operation, no PSA should be detectable, since there is no prostate to produce the antigen. If PSA levels do rise, it generally indicates a recurrence. In these cases, radiation therapy and/or hormone therapy is prescribed.

With respect to PSA, the doctor monitors three different factors: whether PSA levels have increased; how long after the operation this occurs; and how long it takes for PSA levels to double (in other words, PSA velocity). The less time it takes, the higher the risk of recurrence, and the more aggressive the recurrence will be. For example, if PSA levels begin rising eight months after the operation and double in six months, the situation is much more worrisome than if PSA levels begin to rise three years after surgery and take a year to double.

After five years of remission (that is, with no reappearance of the cancer), the risk of future recurrence is very low.

TWO PEOPLE'S STORIES

Name: William	**Age:** 71 years old

Occupation: Retired accountant

William is still alert and in good shape, with no known medical conditions other than localized prostate cancer that is at stage T2 and scores 7 (grades 3 + 4) on the Gleason scale. William's PSA level is 10. Relating his family history, William mentions that his parents died at the ages of 98 and 99. The doctor determines that William probably has a similar life expectancy and presents the three treatment options—active surveillance, radical prostatectomy and radiation therapy—explaining the benefits and drawbacks of each. William opts for radical prostatectomy to maximize his chances of long-term recovery.

Name: John	**Age:** 67 years old

Occupation: Retired math teacher

John is 67 years old and divorced. The doctor informs him that he is suffering from prostate cancer with a stage T2 tumour scoring 7 (3 + 4) on the Gleason scale and PSA testing at 8 ng/mL. According to the Partin table analysis, there is a 46 percent chance the cancer has extended beyond the prostate, but only a 9 percent risk it has affected the seminal vesicles and a 2 percent chance it has spread to the pelvic nodes. John is told that because the risk that the cancer has spread is quite high, he might need other treatments in addition to surgery. The doctor also informs him that the nodes will not be removed, since there is such a low risk that they are affected. The Kattan nomograms are then used to calculate the risk of recurrence after five years, and John learns he has an 85 percent chance of being cured with surgery as his only treatment.

RADIATION THERAPY

External beam radiation therapy

The goal of radiation therapy is to destroy cancerous prostate cells by exposing them to ionizing (radioactive) rays. This treatment, used when the cancer is confined to the prostate, is often very effective. If the cancer seems aggressive, hormone therapy is sometimes prescribed for the months preceding and following radiation therapy (see "Hormone therapy" later in this chapter).

The benefits of radiation are gradual and cumulative. Cell death continues for several months after the treatment is finished, so it is often necessary to wait as long as a year before results can be evaluated. Radiation therapy has become much more precise over the last few years. The standard treatment now in most hospitals is known as "3-D conformal radiation therapy" or "intensity-modulated radiation therapy."

CANCER IN OLDER MEN IS STILL SERIOUS

Prostate cancer is not "worse" in younger men than in older men. While many people believe that cancer cells multiply more quickly in men in their fifties because their metabolism is faster than that of older men, this is not true. The same type of cancer (i.e., the same grade and stage) will progress the same way, no matter what the age of the patient. Indeed, if the type of cancer were the only consideration, treatment would be the same too. The differences in the type of therapy followed by younger and older patients are explained by their varying life expectancies, medical histories and personal choices.

Powerful computers and tomographic scans (CT or CAT scans) generate a more exact, three-dimensional picture of the prostate (Figure ❸). These images enable increased precision when administering the radiation, which maximizes the impact on cancer cells and reduces the negative effects of radiation exposure on the surrounding tissues. The thin radiation beams are directed at the prostate in the lower abdomen. The seminal vesicles are also targeted, as this is where cancer cells often migrate first.

One session of radiation therapy lasts only two to four minutes. It is usually painless and requires no anesthesia whatsoever; for the patient, the experience is similar to having an X-ray. There are generally 35 sessions in all—one session a day, five days a week for seven weeks—and no hospitalization is required. Because the sessions are frequent, the areas to be exposed to radiation are marked on the skin, like little tattoos that last as long as the treatment. Researchers are currently studying the possibility and effectiveness of a treatment regime that would take half the time but deliver stronger doses of radiation.

Although the beams are very precise, it is next to impossible to avoid touching the erectile nerves and healthy cells of the rectum and bladder near the prostate. Radiation therapy is therefore administered at low doses over several sessions (this is also done to avoid as many complications as possible). This allows healthy cells to recover and survive, while the cancerous cells eventually disappear. The urethra, which intersects the prostate, is made of extremely resistant tissue and is barely affected by the radiation.

Side effects of external beam radiation therapy

External beam radiation therapy causes a number of side effects, including fatigue (many patients need a nap during the day), cutaneous (skin) reactions in the pubic area (redness) and hair loss in the areas touched by the rays. Note that it does not cause hair loss anywhere else on the body; the patient can rest assured he will not go bald.

The treatment also affects the bladder and rectum, because they are so close to the prostate. Some men therefore

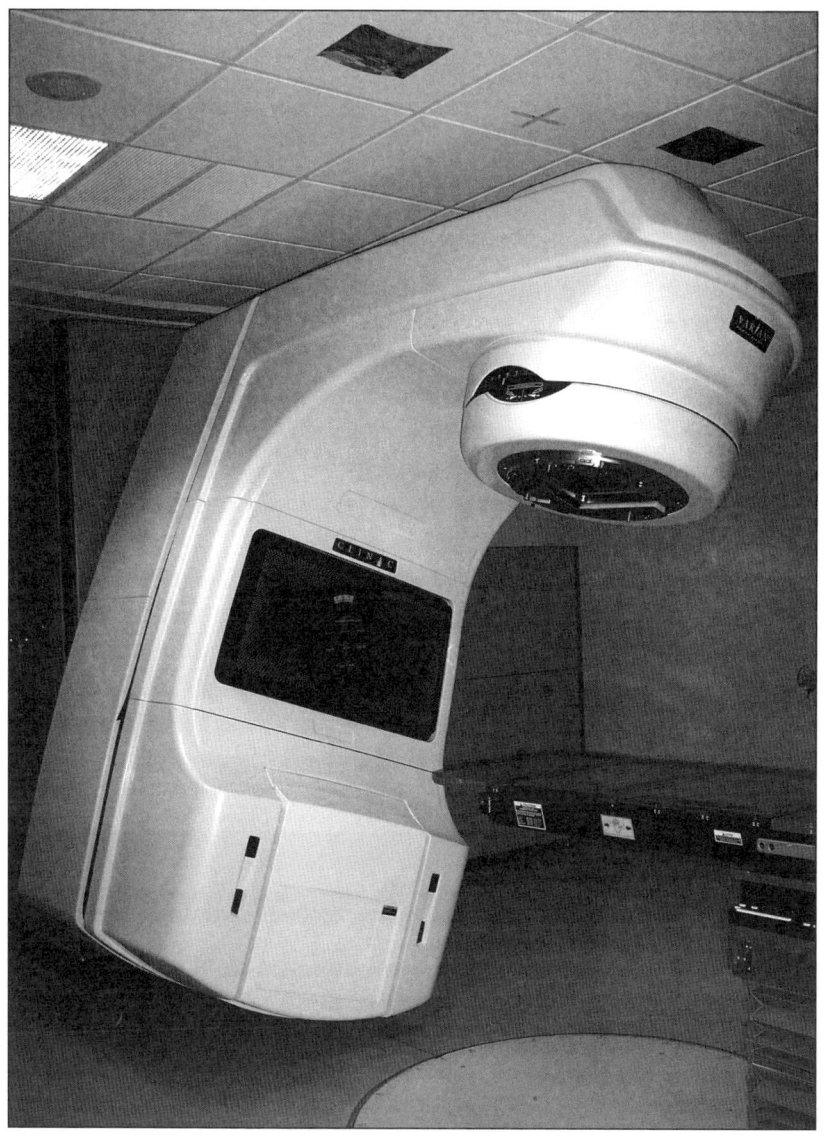

❸ External beam therapy equipment (linear accelerator)

experience a frequent or urgent need to urinate (often disrupting their sleep), blood in the urine, burning with urination, diarrhea, anal irritation or rectal bleeding. The doctor can prescribe medication to alleviate these adverse effects.

Most side effects disappear gradually over the year following treatment.

Long-term complications of external beam radiation therapy

In 5 to 10 percent of cases, intestinal and urinary function does not return to normal after treatment is complete. Medications (such as cortisone to reduce anal inflammation) and muscle relaxants can help ease these side effects.

In 40 to 60 percent of patients, the rays cause permanent erectile dysfunction. Unlike other side effects, however, erectile difficulties develop gradually, because cell death happens slowly and progressively. Erection capacity remains intact at first, but diminishes over several months (or sometimes even years) following treatment. There are, however, a number of treatments available to help men regain their erectile capacity and enjoy a satisfying sex life again (see Chapter 6).

DOES THE PENIS REALLY GET SMALLER?

In rare cases, patients who have undergone radical prostatectomy or external beam radiation therapy have the impression their penis has become shorter. While this is technically not the case, the penis does sometimes retract if it has not become erect for a long period of time due to the lack of blood flow. Recent studies suggest that drugs such as Cialis, Levitra or Viagra should be used on a continuous basis very soon after surgery to accelerate the recovery of erections and reduce the risk of the penis retracting.

Radiation therapy also "dries out" the prostate. In many cases, this means the gland stops producing the substances that make up semen and nourish sperm cells (see "The Functions of the Prostate" in Chapter 1), resulting in a significant decrease in the amount of ejaculate. In addition, most men who undergo radiation therapy become infertile. It should be emphasized, however, that the ability to achieve orgasm remains intact, since it is controlled by nerves located far from the prostate. The man's sex drive is also preserved, unless he undergoes hormone therapy (see "Hormone therapy" below).

Results and medical follow-up of external beam radiation therapy

As in the case of radical prostatectomy, it is impossible to estimate the average success rate of radiation therapy. The odds of a cure vary widely from person to person because of individual differences in the grade of the tumour, the degree to which the cancer has spread and pre-treatment PSA levels. In general, the less severe these three factors are, the better the patient's chances of a complete cure.

For example, there is a relatively low risk of recurrence for a man with PSA levels under 10 ng/mL and a stage T1 or T2 tumour that scores 6 (grades 3 + 3) on the Gleason scale. On the other hand, the risk of recurrence (either localized or distant) is quite high for a man presenting any one of the following signs before treatment: PSA levels over 20, a stage T3 tumour or a tumour scoring 8 or more on the Gleason scale. In the latter case, the doctor would probably immediately recommend that hormone therapy precede and follow radiation treatment.

Every three to six months, a rectal exam is performed and PSA level is measured to monitor the patient's status. PSA levels should begin to drop in the months following the start of treatment and may continue to do so for as long as a year after treatment ends. The lower they fall, the greater the chances that the cancer is fully under control. Since radiation therapy does not destroy 100 percent of the prostate cells, PSA levels will generally not fall all the way to 0 ng/mL; in most cases, they decrease to less than 1 ng/mL and remain stable.

If PSA readings begin to rise, the doctor will keep a close watch on how long it takes for them to double. The less time it takes, the greater the risk of recurrence and the more aggressive it will be.

When the patient begins to experience erectile difficulties, the doctor will prescribe medication to help him regain his erectile capacity (see Chapter 6).

The patient is monitored for at least five years after radiation therapy. If the cancer is still in remission by the end of this period, it will likely remain so, but annual follow-up appointments are still scheduled as a precaution.

Brachytherapy (permanent or temporary radioactive implant)

External beams are not the only way to administer radiation therapy. Low dose brachytherapy—also known as seed implant therapy—involves placing small pellets containing radioactive materials directly into the prostate (Figure ❹). These pellets are known as seeds, and each one is about the size of a grain of rice. This treatment is most effective in cancers that are not particularly aggressive—that is, when PSA levels are lower than 10, the tumour is stage T1 or T2 and the Gleason score is no more than 6 (3 + 3) (note that all three of these conditions must be met for best results).

The size of the man's prostate before treatment is also important. Brachytherapy causes the prostate to swell temporarily; if the gland is already large because of the cancer, further enlargement could compress the urethra, preventing the patient from urinating and causing quite a bit of pain. The doctor might prescribe a three-month cycle of hormone therapy before radiation treatment to reduce prostate size (see "Hormone therapy" below). The patient must not have severe lower urinary tract symptoms (LUTS or so-called prostatism) caused by the prostate obstructing the

CHAPTER 4 – TREATMENT OF LOCALIZED PROSTATE CANCER

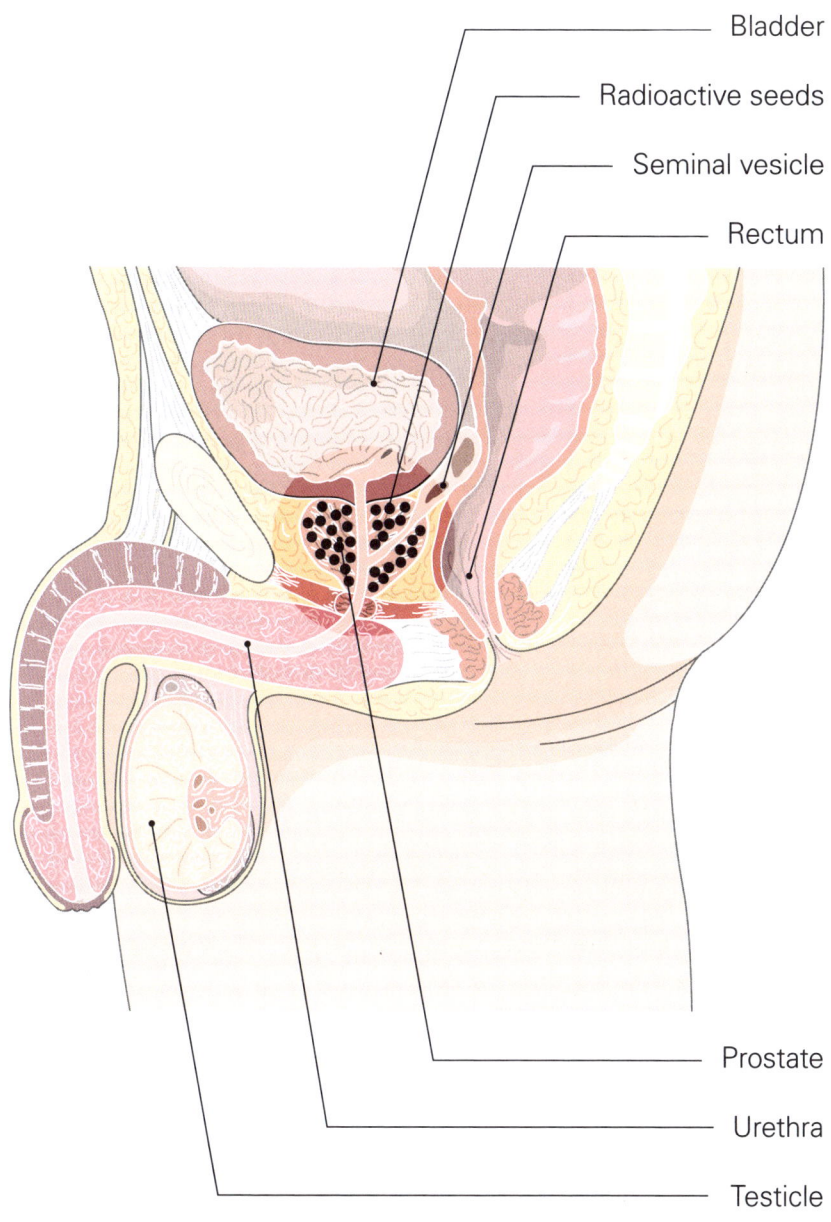

❹ Brachytherapy

bladder (see Chapter 1), as radiation therapy will only worsen these symptoms.

One of the main advantages of brachytherapy is that it requires only one brief visit to the hospital, whereas external beam radiation therapy involves approximately thirty separate treatments. Brachytherapy also has a much shorter recovery time than radical prostatectomy, since there is no operative stress and no period of convalescence.

The doctor first uses transrectal ultrasonography (TRUS, see Chapter 3) to get a clear image of the prostate and chart the placement of the radioactive seeds. The seeds are then inserted into the gland through the perineum (the area between the testicles and the anus) using a thin rod made of lead to contain the radioactivity. A few hospitals offer the option of performing the procedure using only a local anesthetic, but most patients find this too uncomfortable and choose either general or epidural (waist down) anesthesia. Brachytherapy does not usually require hospitalization.

The number of seeds required depends on the size of the prostate (on average, about fifty are inserted). To be effective, the seeds must be spread evenly throughout the gland. The seeds are too small for the patient to feel, let alone to cause any discomfort.

Once inserted, the seeds cannot be removed, but the patient should not worry as they remain radioactive for a limited period of time (usually under a year) and do not cause any damage to the body. They have been known to become dislodged from the gland, but this is extremely rare.

In North America, brachytherapy is increasing in popularity because it is much less stressful and traumatic than traditional radiation therapy or radical prostatectomy. However, the treatment is not indicated in cases of aggressive cancer, and its effectiveness in comparison with external beam radiation therapy or radical prostatectomy is unknown. Furthermore, it is a very expensive treatment and therefore not available in every treatment centre.

Another form of brachytherapy is high-dose rate (HDR) temporary brachytherapy . In this case, thin rods are inserted into the prostate much the same as in seed implants, but they are left in place only for the time needed to send a short burst of radiation (usually in one to three shots). This serves as a boost to external beam radiation and allows a higher dose of radiation to be given in less time and with fewer side effects. Studies are ongoing to determine if this will lead to better cancer control in patients at higher risk of recurrence.

Side effects of brachytherapy
Piercing the prostate in several places causes the gland to swell. This can lead to problems such as pain with urination, an urgent need to urinate, difficulty urinating and burning with urination. The doctor can prescribe medication to alleviate these side effects. In some cases, the treatment results in complete blockage and a total inability to urinate. If this occurs despite preventive measures, a temporary catheter is inserted to empty the bladder. This symptom will gradually disappear on its own.

Side effects also include diarrhea, anal irritation and rectal bleeding, which last an average of three to four months. The doctor can prescribe medication to alleviate these effects.

Fatigue, skin reactions in the pubic area and hair loss are much less pronounced with brachytherapy than with the standard therapy.

Long-term complications of brachytherapy
Brachytherapy causes permanent erectile dysfunction in 20 to 50 percent of men. As with external radiation therapy, erectile difficulties do not develop immediately but arise gradually over the months following treatment. Once the patient begins to notice a problem, the doctor prescribes medication to help him regain his erectile capacity (see Chapter 6).

Like external beam radiation therapy, brachytherapy also "dries out" the prostate. The gland therefore stops producing the substances that make up semen (see Chapter 1), and patients can expect a significant decrease in the amount of ejaculate. Most men who undergo this treatment also become infertile. The nerves controlling orgasm capacity, however, are located far from the prostate and are therefore not affected. Sex drive also remains intact, unless the patient has undergone hormone therapy as well (see "Hormone therapy" below).

In very rare cases, brachytherapy can cause long-term urinary incontinence. For more information concerning urinary and erectile problems and solutions, see Chapter 6.

Results and medical follow-up of brachytherapy
As in the case of other treatment methods, it is impossible to estimate average success rate for brachytherapy. The odds of success vary widely from person to person because of individual differences in the grade of the tumour, the degree to which the cancer has spread and PSA levels. The less severe these three factors are, the better the patient's chances of a complete cure.

Every three to six months, a rectal exam is performed and PSA level is measured to monitor the patient's status. PSA levels should decrease in the months after treatment begins and may continue dropping after it finishes. The lower PSA levels fall, the better the odds that the cancer is fully under control. Even if everything is still fine after five years, annual follow-up visits are scheduled as a precaution.

If PSA readings begin to rise, the doctor will keep a close watch on how long it takes for them to double. The less time it takes, the greater the risk of recurrence and the more aggressive it will be. However, because brachytherapy is usually prescribed for men with cancers that are not particularly aggressive, the risk of recurrence tends to be fairly low.

Because this is a relatively new technique, there is less information available about its long-term results, particularly in comparison with external beam radiation therapy or radical prostatectomy.

HIGH-DOSE RATE (HDR) BRACHYTHERAPY

This form of brachytherapy involves delivering significantly higher doses of radiation through radioactive sources placed temporarily in the prostate.

The surgical intervention is performed under spinal or general anesthesia and is similar to that required for standard brachytherapy; however, instead of seeds, about 12 to 15 thin rods are inserted into the prostate through the perineum. After surgery, the patient is moved to a special room where radioactive rays are directed through the rods. Once the full dose has been delivered, the rods are withdrawn.

While HDR brachytherapy is not effective when used alone, research is ongoing to determine if it may improve cure rates in conjunction with external beam radiation therapy. It may allow the number of radiation treatments to be cut in half, although the effectiveness and long-term side effects of HDR brachytherapy are still unknown. Short-term side effects appear to be very similar to those of external beam radiation therapy.

TWO PEOPLE'S STORIES

Name: Eric   **Age:** 73 years old

Occupation: Retired journalist

Eric has had coronary bypass surgery. His cancer seems fairly aggressive at stage T2 and scoring 8 (grades 4 + 4) on the Gleason scale. His PSA level is 20.

Eric wants a treatment that will help control his disease and give him hope for recovery. Given his age and history of heart disease, he and his doctor choose radiation therapy rather than surgery. Adding hormone therapy to radiation for two or three years will help him control the disease better in the long term and increase his chances of survival.

Name: Paul   **Age:** 56 years old

Occupation: Mail carrier

Paul is in excellent shape. However, he recently discovered that he has relatively aggressive localized prostate cancer that is at stage T1 and scores 7 (grades 3 + 4) on the Gleason scale. His PSA level is 9.

Paul's doctor suggests radical prostatectomy, adding that he may also need radiation therapy depending on what is discovered during the operation.

Paul doesn't hesitate. He is about to become a grandfather for the first time, and he wants to see his grandchildren grow up. He is aware of the side effects and complications of treatment but reckons they are a small price to pay for being able to continue enjoying his family in the years to come.

FOCAL THERAPY

Traditionally, men with localized prostate cancer are offered either active surveillance or treatment with surgery and/or radiation. Although surgery and radiation have comparable long-term survival rates, they can be associated with significant morbidity, including incontinence and erectile problems. On the other hand, active surveillance is not always acceptable to men with prostate cancer and their doctors. Focal therapy aims to offer a compromise between these two options, because it is less invasive. Two focal therapeutic techniques, HIFU (high-intensity focused ultrasound) and cryotherapy are currently being evaluated more extensively. At the present time, however, neither can be considered a viable alternative to the standard treatment options for localized prostate cancer.

High-intensity focused ultrasound (HIFU)

High-intensity focused ultrasound (HIFU) is a procedure in which a probe inserted into the rectum emits a focused sound wave at the prostate, raising the temperature and destroying cells. The treatment usually takes one to three hours depending on the size of the prostate.

HIFU has been used for several years in Europe and is now available in Canada. HIFU is not available in the United States because the FDA (Food and Drug Administration) has made no decision as to its safety or efficacy in the treatment of prostate cancer. Interest in this treatment is growing, and research is ongoing to determine its efficacy and the patients most likely to benefit from it.

Cryotherapy

A recent alternative to surgery and radiation therapy that is used in some centres in Canada is cryotherapy, or freezing of the prostate gland, also called cryoablation. This is done through the perineum (between the testicles and the anus), like brachytherapy. Catheters are placed within the prostate gland and the temperature is lowered to extremely cold temperatures that cause cell death. The results to date are encouraging in patients with persistent local disease that radiation therapy has failed to control, and cryotherapy has recently become a viable alternative for some patients. Although it is still too early to assess the long-term efficacy of this treatment, short-term results appear comparable to those of external beam radiation therapy in selected patients. The future will show if this type of treatment will become another option for patients with localized prostate cancer. Possible complications of cryotherapy include erectile dysfunction, incontinence and rectal injury.

HORMONE THERAPY

In some cases, hormone therapy to eliminate androgens, also called androgen deprivation therapy (ADT), is recommended for three to eight months before radiation therapy (external beam radiation therapy or brachytherapy) to reduce the size of the tumour and make it easier to treat. This is known as neoadjuvant hormone therapy. Some doctors recommend this treatment before radical prostatectomy to make it easier to remove the gland, although this is still an experimental approach and to date has not been demonstrated to increase the chances of cure.

Adjuvant hormone therapy is prescribed after radiation therapy or a radical prostatectomy when, according to the grade and stage of the tumour and PSA levels, it appears that the cancer cells may have spread away from the prostate area. Note that this does not necessarily mean the cancer has metastasized; it may be that the cancer cells were not completely removed at the time of prostatectomy but survived the initial treatment and remained undetected in the body, increasing the risk of recurrence. Hormone therapy is a systemic treatment (i.e., it acts on the entire body) and can treat these cells immediately. It is prescribed for one to three years.

CHAPTER 4 – TREATMENT OF LOCALIZED PROSTATE CANCER

Both neoadjuvant (before radiation therapy/radical prostatectomy) and adjuvant (after radiation therapy/radical prostatectomy) hormone therapies involve regular injections of LH-RH (luteinizing hormone-releasing hormone) analogs or antagonists. These synthetic compounds imitate naturally produced LH-RH and prevent the testicles from producing testosterone. As testosterone helps cultivate prostate cancer (see Chapter 2), impeding its production reduces the size of the tumour and the prostate gland.

Hormone therapy cannot cure cancer by itself, but it can slow the progression of the disease. In some patients, particularly those with shorter life expectancies, it is the sole treatment.

Hormone therapy as a treatment for localized prostate cancer began in the 1990s, and there is still no clear consensus regarding its optimal use. The only thing clearly established is that it is recommended for locally advanced cancers (stage T3 tumours scoring 8 or more on the Gleason scale and PSA levels of 20 ng/mL or more) in conjunction with radiation therapy. The data available on other types of cases, however, are not clear enough for doctors to determine the therapy's effectiveness or to ascertain which patients should receive it, when it should be prescribed or for how long. Without this basic framework, doctors have only their individual judgment to rely on. It is very likely, however, that there will be some progress in this field over the next few years.

If nodal metastasis exists (discovered during surgery or suspected using the Partin tables), radical prostatectomy or radiation therapy is usually not enough, and long-term hormone therapy is indicated to control the disease throughout the entire body (see Chapter 5).

Side effects of hormone therapy

Hormone therapy indirectly causes erectile dysfunction by lowering testosterone levels and therefore the sex drive. With no libido, the patient finds it very difficult to achieve an erection, and, unfortunately, medications available to treat erectile dysfunction have little benefit in such cases.

Hormone therapy can also cause hot flashes, anemia, fatigue, mood swings, weight gain, loss of muscle mass and, in some cases, breast tissue growth. The doctor can prescribe medication to alleviate hot flashes, but there is no treatment for any of the other side effects.

If the hormone therapy is relatively short (under a year), side effects generally disappear and the man's sex drive returns. His breasts also stop increasing in size, although they will not get smaller again.

Long-term complications of hormone therapy

The longer a patient takes hormone therapy, the greater the risk of permanent side effects. In addition, after one year of treatment, patients may begin to experience bone loss and could eventually develop osteoporosis, although medications are available to prevent or treat this condition. After two years of therapy, many men must learn to live with the fact that the complications (including loss of sex drive) may become permanent. However, most accept this consequence fairly easily, since the treatment significantly slows the progression of the disease and potentially adds years to their lives.

Recently there have been studies suggesting that hormone therapy may increase the risk of developing diabetes and possibly heart disease. Even though this has not been clearly demonstrated, it must be considered when weighing the pros and cons of hormone therapy. In most patients with high-risk disease, the benefits of hormone therapy outweigh the risks.

Results and medical follow-up of hormone therapy

Every three to six months, PSA measurements are taken and occasionally digital rectal exams are performed to monitor the patient's status. The lower PSA levels fall, the better the chances that the cancer is fully under control. The objective, however, is to stabilize PSA levels not to reach 0 ng/mL (although if the patient has also undergone a radical prostatectomy, PSA should be undetectable).

As long as PSA levels remain stable, the cancer is considered to be in remission. If they begin to rise, the doctor will keep a close watch on how long it takes them to double. The less time it takes, the higher the risk of recurrence and the more aggressive it will be. If the cancer recurs, that means it is castration-resistant (formerly called hormone-refractory), and the patient may have to turn to the treatments described in the next chapter.

PREDICTIVE TOOLS

Partin tables

At the end of the 1990s, Dr. Alan W. Partin of Johns Hopkins Medical Center in the United States developed a table (or scale) to help determine the extent of a localized prostate cancer at the time of diagnosis for the purposes of radical prostatectomy. He gathered data from thousands of patients who had undergone both radical prostatectomy and pelvic lymphadenectomy (removal of the pelvic lymph nodes, described in Chapter 3).

Dr. Partin discovered that by combining the malignancy grade according to the Gleason scale, the stage of the tumour (its size as perceived in a digital rectal exam) and the patient's PSA level (higher measurements indicating an increased likelihood of advanced cancer), the disease could be assessed more accurately, giving the doctor a better idea of what to expect during surgery and which treatments would be optimal.

The Partin tables are also used to evaluate whether the pelvic lymph nodes have been affected. This information can affect the surgical protocol; that is, it can influence whether the doctor decides to remove nodes for analysis before proceeding with the prostatectomy.

The Partin tables are quite reliable and many doctors use them regularly. Of course, the patient also appreciates having a more precise idea of the state of the cancer upon diagnosis, but he is certainly more interested in knowing his chances of a complete cure. This is where the Kattan nomograms come in.

PARTIN'S TABLES

PSA Range (ng/mL)	Pathologic Stage	Biopsy Gleason Score			
		5-6	3 + 4 = 7	4 + 3 = 7	8-10
Clinical Stage T1c (non-palpable. PSA elevated)					
0-2.5	Organ confined	93 (91-95)*	82 (76-87)	73 (64-80)	77 (65-85)
	Extraprostatic extension	6 (5-8)	14 (10-18)	20 (14-28)	16 (11-24)
	Seminal vesicle**	0 (0-1)	2 (0-5)	2 (0-5)	3 (0-8)
	Lymph node**	0 (0-1)	2 (0-6)	4 (1-12)	3 (1-12)
2.6-4.0	Organ confined	88 (86-90)	72 (67-76)	61 (54-68)	66 (57-74)
	Extraprostatic extension	11 (10-13)	23 (19-27)	33 (27-39)	26 (19-34)
	Seminal vesicle	1 (0-1)	4 (2-7)	5 (2-8)	7 (3-13)
	Lymph node	0 (0-0)	1 (0-1)	1 (0-3)	1 (0-3)
4.1-6.0	Organ confined	83 (81-85)	63 (59-67)	51 (45-56)	55 (46-64)
	Extraprostatic extension	16 (14-17)	30 (26-33)	40 (34-45)	32 (25-40)
	Seminal vesicle	1 (1-1)	6 (4-8)	7 (4-10)	10 (6-15)
	Lymph node	0 (0-0)	2 (1-3)	3 (1-6)	3 (1-6)
6.1-10.0	Organ confined	81 (79-83)	59 (54-64)	47 (41-53)	51 (41-59)
	Extraprostatic extension	18 (16-19)	32 (27-36)	42 (36-47)	34 (26-42)
	Seminal vesicle	1 (1-2)	8 (6-11)	8 (5-12)	12 (8-19)
	Lymph node	0 (0-0)	1 (1-3)	3 (1-5)	3 (1-5)
>10.0	Organ confined	70 (66-74)	42 (37-48)	30 (25-36)	34 (26-42)
	Extraprostatic extension	27 (23-30)	40 (35-45)	48 (40-55)	39 (31-48)
	Seminal vesicle	2 (2-3)	12 (8-16)	11 (7-17)	17 (10-25)
	Lymph node	1 (0-1)	6 (3-9)	10 (5-17)	9 (4-17)
Clinical Stage T2a (palpable < ½ of one lobe)					
0-2.5	Organ confined	88 (84-90)	70 (63-77)	58 (48-67)	63 (51-74)
	Extraprostatic extension	12 (9-15)	24 (18-30)	32 (24-41)	26 (18-36)
	Seminal vesicle	0 (0-1)	2 (0-6)	3 (0-7)	4 (0-10)
	Lymph node	0 (0-1)	3 (1-9)	7 (1-17)	6 (1-16)
2.6-4.0	Organ confined	79 (75-82)	57 (51-63)	45 (38-52)	50 (40-59)
	Extraprostatic extension	20 (17-24)	37 (31-42)	48 (40-55)	40 (30-50)
	Seminal vesicle	1 (0-1)	5 (3-9)	5 (3-10)	8 (4-15)
	Lymph node	0 (0-0)	1 (1-2)	2 (0-5)	2 (0-4)
4.1-6.0	Organ confined	71 (67-75)	47 (41-52)	34 (28-41)	39 (31-48)
	Extraprostatic extension	27 (23-31)	44 (39-49)	54 (47-60)	46 (37-54)
	Seminal vesicle	1 (1-2)	7 (4-10)	7 (4-11)	11 (6-17)
	Lymph node	0 (0-1)	2 (1-4)	5 (2-8)	4 (2-9)

CHAPTER 4 – TREATMENT OF LOCALIZED PROSTATE CANCER

PSA Range (ng/mL)	Pathologic Stage	Biopsy Gleason Score			
		5-6	3 + 4 = 7	4 + 3 = 7	8-10
6.1-10.0	Organ confined	68 (74-72)	43 (38-48)	31 (26-37)	36 (27-44)
	Extraprostatic extension	29 (26-33)	46 (41-51)	56 (49-62)	47 (37-56)
	Seminal vesicle	2 (1-3)	9 (6-13)	9 (5-14)	13 (8-20)
	Lymph node	0 (0-1)	2 (1-4)	4 (2-8)	4 (1-8)
>10.0	Organ confined	54 (49-60)	28 (23-33)	18 (14-23)	21 (15-28)
	Extraprostatic extension	41 (35-46)	52 (46-59)	57 (48-66)	49 (39-59)
	Seminal vesicle	3 (2-5)	12 (7-18)	11 (6-17)	17 (9-25)
	Lymph node	1 (0-3)	7 (3-14)	13 (6-24)	12 (5-22)

Clinical Stage T2b (palpable ≥ ½ of lobe) or T2c (palpable both lobes)

PSA Range (ng/mL)	Pathologic Stage	5-6	3 + 4 = 7	4 + 3 = 7	8-10
0-2.5	Organ confined	84 (78-89)	59 (47-70)	44 (31-58)	49 (32-65)
	Extraprostatic extension	14 (9-19)	24 (16-33)	29 (19-42)	24 (14-36)
	Seminal vesicle	1 (0-3)	6 (0-14)	6 (0-14)	8 (0-21)
	Lymph node	1 (0-3)	10 (2-25)	19 (4-40)	17 (3-42)
2.6-4.0	Organ confined	74 (68-80)	47 (39-56)	36 (27-45)	39 (28-50)
	Extraprostatic extension	23 (18-29)	37 (28-45)	46 (36-55)	37 (27-48)
	Seminal vesicle	2 (0-5)	13 (7-21)	13 (7-22)	19 (9-32)
	Lymph node	0 (0-1)	3 (0-7)	5 (0-14)	4 (0-13)
4.1-6.0	Organ confined	66 (59-72)	36 (29-43)	25 (19-32)	27 (19-37)
	Extraprostatic extension	30 (24-36)	41 (33-47)	47 (38-55)	38 (28-48)
	Seminal vesicle	4 (2-6)	16 (10-23)	15 (9-23)	22 (13-33)
	Lymph node	1 (0-2)	7 (3-12)	13 (6-21)	11 (4-23)
6.1-10.0	Organ confined	62 (55-68)	32 (26-38)	22 (17-29)	24 (17-33)
	Extraprostatic extension	32 (26-38)	41 (33-49)	47 (38-56)	38 (29-48)
	Seminal vesicle	5 (3-8)	20 (13-28)	19 (11-28)	27 (16-39)
	Lymph node	1 (0-2)	6 (3-11)	11 (5-19)	10 (3-20)
>10.0	Organ confined	46 (39-53)	18 (13-24)	11 (7-15)	12 (7-18)
	Extraprostatic extension	41 (34-50)	40 (31-51)	40 (30-52)	33 (22-46)
	Seminal vesicle	7 (4-12)	23 (15-33)	19 (10-29)	28 (16-42)
	Lymph node	5 (2-8)	18 (9-30)	29 (15-44)	26 (12-44)

** Values are percent probability (95% confidence interval) of a given pathologic stage.
** Affected

Data source: Updated Nomogram to Predict Pathologic Stage of Prostate Cancer Given Prostate-Specific Antigen Level, Clinical Stage, and Biopsy Gleason Score (Partin Tables) Based on Cases from 2000 to 2005, *Urology, 2007*, with permission from Elsevier

Kattan nomograms

In 1999, Dr. Mike Kattan, an American statistician specializing in medicine, created a scale to compute the risk of recurrence within five years of surgery or radiation therapy based on the rise in PSA after treatment. He decided on five years because the risk of recurrence is low if the cancer has not reappeared by then.

The Kattan nomograms take into account the same data as the Partin tables, namely, the grade and stage of the tumour and PSA levels at the time of diagnosis. A calculation is then performed to establish the probability of PSA levels rising within five years of treatment (if they remain at 0 ng/mL, the disease is fully under control). The higher the probability, the lower the chances of a complete cure. The risk of recurrence can help determine whether additional treatments are required.

Albertsen life tables

In 1999, Dr. Peter Albertsen, an American urologist specializing in epidemiology, developed a scale to calculate the risk for patients receiving no treatment at all of dying from prostate cancer in the next 15 years compared to their risk of dying from other causes. The tables, which take into account the patient's age and the grade of the tumour, resulted from 20 years of follow-up of patients who never underwent active treatment for their prostate cancer.

Doctors use the tables when they are unsure what type of treatment the patient should follow given his age and the tumour's aggressiveness, or when the patient wants to know the probable outcome if he decides to forgo treatment. Fifteen years might seem like a distant projection, but prostate cancer often progresses quite slowly. The slow development of the disease also explains why the patient's general state of health (and therefore his chances of dying from other causes) is also considered when choosing treatment.

CHAPTER 4 – TREATMENT OF LOCALIZED PROSTATE CANCER

ONE PERSON'S STORY

Name: Richard   **Age:** 55 years old

Occupation: Electrician

Richard is married and works for a large company as an electrician. His cancer scores 8 (grades 4 + 4) on the Gleason scale. He has a stage T3 tumour and a PSA level of 15 ng/mL. Partin table analysis indicates there is only a 6 percent chance the cancer is still confined to the prostate and a 26 percent chance it has spread to the pelvic nodes. The CT scan suggests his cancer has spread to the lymph nodes in the pelvis.

Given the lymph node metastasis, the chances of a cure are slim, even with surgery. In addition, Richard would like to minimize the risk of complications. He and his doctor decide on hormone therapy and radiation therapy.

These two therapies together should help to control the disease in the long term. Richard remains optimistic even if a cure is unlikely, since he is well aware that there are options if the cancer recurs.

KEY POINTS TO REMEMBER

- The treatment of localized prostate cancer is determined on the basis of three factors: the grade of the tumour, the stage of the tumour and PSA levels. These elements guide the assessment of the disease and of the chances of survival in the coming years. The doctor also considers the patient's age, life expectancy, family history and medical history.

- In cases where the tumour remains confined to the prostate, either radical prostatectomy or radiation therapy is often sufficient treatment. Indeed, both options are quite effective and have equal cure rates for the five- to ten-year period after treatment. After 10 years, recurrences are slightly less common in men who have undergone a radical prostatectomy.

- In cases of locally advanced cancer, treatment might involve a combination of radical prostatectomy, radiation therapy and possibly hormone therapy. If the pelvic nodes have been affected, surgery or radiation is usually insufficient and hormone therapy is most often prescribed to control the disease throughout the entire body. If hormone therapy is begun before bone metastasis takes place, the chances of survival are significantly higher.

- It is impossible to calculate the exact success rate for any of these treatments. Every patient reacts differently because of individual variations in the grade of the tumour, the degree to which the cancer has spread and PSA levels before treatment. The lower all these are, the better the chances of a cure.

- When patients are diagnosed with localized and apparently slow-growing cancers, watchful waiting or active surveillance may be offered depending on the circumstances. There is usually enough time for the doctor to intervene with some form of treatment if the disease begins to progress more rapidly.

CHAPTER 4 – TREATMENT OF LOCALIZED PROSTATE CANCER

- Erectile dysfunction affects approximately 50 percent of men who undergo radical prostatectomy with the erectile nerves preserved and almost 100 percent of those whose nerves could not be spared. External beam radiation therapy causes permanent erectile difficulties in 40 to 60 percent of cases. With brachytherapy (also known as seed implant therapy), the risk is 20 to 50 percent.

- Thankfully, there are treatments for erectile dysfunction (see Chapter 6) that allow most men to regain their erectile capacity and enjoy a satisfying sex life.

- Hormone therapy indirectly causes erectile dysfunction by lowering testosterone levels, resulting in a loss of sex drive which begins in the first few weeks of treatment. If the therapy does not last too long (for example, less than a year), the side effects will usually disappear on their own.

- Stress incontinence is a complication affecting 10 percent of men who have had a prostatectomy; 1 to 5 percent will suffer from significant urinary incontinence. External beam radiation therapy causes permanent urinary problems in only 5 to 10 percent of men, brachytherapy causes this effect in even fewer cases, and hormone therapy has no effect on continence whatsoever.

- Every three to six months, PSA measurements are taken and digital rectal exams may be performed to monitor the patient's status. PSA levels should diminish and remain stable after treatment. An increase in PSA level indicates a probable recurrence.

CHAPTER 5
TREATMENT OF ADVANCED PROSTATE CANCER

Advanced prostate cancer exists in different forms: localized cancer recurring after initial treatment, locally advanced non-metastatic cancer, metastatic cancer and metastatic or non-metastatic cancer recurring despite hormone therapy.

In most cases, the best treatment for advanced prostate cancer is still hormone therapy (elimination of androgens). However, recent studies have shown that chemotherapy can be useful in cases of castration-resistant prostate cancer (CRPC), formerly known as hormone-refractrory prostate cancer (cancer progresses during hormone therapy). Even if a cure is not always possible, it is important to remain optimistic. We are making progress in changing prostate cancer from a life-threatening disease to a chronic and controllable disease.

HORMONE THERAPY

In the early 1940s, Dr. Charles Brenton Huggins, an American surgeon born in Canada and working in Chicago, discovered that prostate cancer is dependent on male hormones for growth and that suppressing these hormones induces remission of the disease. This breakthrough profoundly changed the treatment of prostate cancer and earned Dr. Huggins the Nobel Prize for Medicine in 1966.

Testosterone, which originates in the testicles, constitutes 85 to 95 percent of male hormones (also known as androgens). The other 5 to 15 percent is made up of similar hormones secreted by the adrenal glands, located just above the kidneys.

Testosterone secretion is regulated by a mechanism originating in the brain. The hypothalamus produces LH-RH (luteinizing hormone-releasing hormone), triggering the release of LH (luteinizing hormone) by the pituitary gland. LH is then carried through the bloodstream to the testicles to stimulate the production of testosterone (Figure ❶).

The objective of hormone therapy, also called androgen deprivation therapy (ADT), as a treatment for advanced prostate cancer is to prevent the testicles from producing testosterone. This is achieved in one of two ways: physical removal of the testicles (surgical castration) or regular injection of LH-RH analogs (medical castration). Suppressing testosterone inhibits cancer growth, causes symptoms to regress or disappear and can even send metastases into remission, sometimes for years.

"Remission" is not exactly synonymous with "cured," although it does mean the disease is under control. When cancer goes into remission, patients can generally expect to live a long time with a relatively good quality of life.

Orchiectomy (surgical castration)
For several decades, surgical removal of the testicles was the only known treatment for advanced prostate cancer. Orchiectomy—also known as surgical castration—immediately and permanently deprives cancerous prostate cells of testosterone.

CHAPTER 5 – TREATMENT OF ADVANCED PROSTATE CANCER

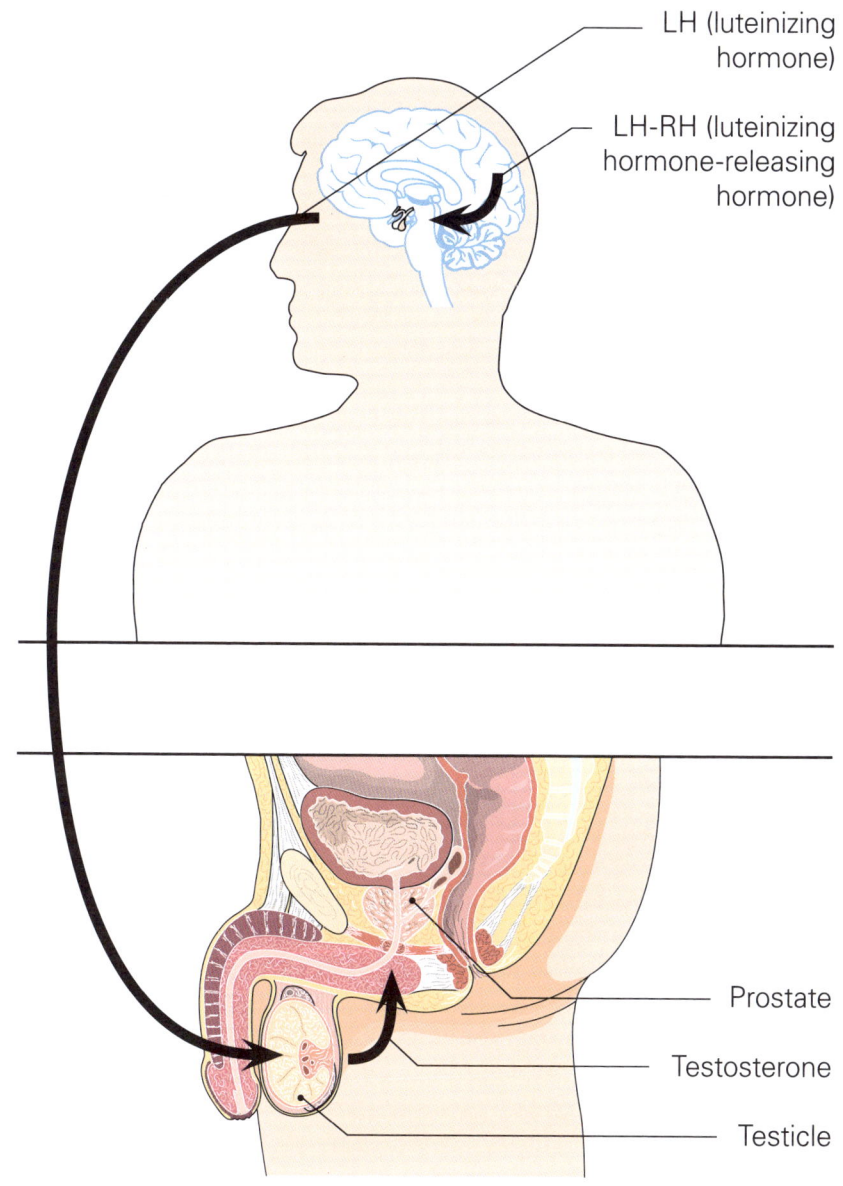

❶ The hormonal pathway

The procedure itself takes approximately 15 minutes and is usually performed under anesthesia, either general or epidural (from the waist down). A small incision is made in the scrotum, and the testicles are removed through this incision. The empty scrotum is then re-sewn, leaving a scar slightly bigger than that caused by a vasectomy. In some cases, patients feel small lumps in the scrotum, caused by scarring at the end of the spermatic cords. In general, the procedure does not require hospitalization, is well tolerated and causes very few complications. Most patients resume their normal routine after two or three weeks.

The first doctors who performed this surgery witnessed astonishing even "miraculous" results. Some patients who had been very ill and confined to hospital were back on their feet and doing much better within 24 hours of the operation. These days, such dramatic transformations rarely occur because the cancer is generally detected long before any symptoms appear.

In addition, surgical removal of the testicles is now performed in only about 1 percent of cases in North America and is presented as an option only when it becomes clear that the patient will need hormone therapy for the rest of his life. In such cases, the one-time procedure can be an alternative to lifelong treatment requiring regular injections.

Today, most men who need hormone therapy take medication in the form of LH-RH analogs.

LH-RH analog therapy (medical castration)

This treatment is known as "medical castration" because it suppresses testosterone production without surgical intervention. It involves administering luteinizing hormone-releasing hormone (LH-RH) analogs (synthetic compounds that imitate the LH-RH produced by the hypothalamus). Paradoxically, LH-RH analog treatment suppresses testosterone production by continuously over-stimulating the pituitary gland. Eventually, the gland becomes exhausted and ceases to produce the luteinizing hormone (LH) altogether, thereby depriving the testicles of the trigger they need to manufacture testosterone.

CHAPTER 5 – TREATMENT OF ADVANCED PROSTATE CANCER

Treatment involves administering regular injections of long-acting LH-RH analogs or antagonists at intervals of one to six months, depending on the drug dose and type (see box, "LH-RH analogs"). The length of treatment is determined by the stage of the disease and ranges from a few months for localized prostate cancers (see Chapter 4) to much longer for advanced cases. Some patients require continuous or intermittent treatment for the rest of their lives (see box, "Continuous or intermittent LH-RH analog therapy?"). Hormone therapy is also a quick-acting pain reliever in very advanced cases of prostate cancer where bone metastasis has occurred.

During the first days of LH-RH analog treatment, the overstimulation of the pituitary gland causes testosterone levels to temporarily increase. In a small percentage of patients, this momentary surge aggravates cancer symptoms. Patients with widespread bone metastasis, for example, run a higher risk of pain or bone fracture during this period.

To spare the patient these heightened symptoms, an additional treatment of non-steroidal anti-androgens (see box, "Anti-androgens") may be prescribed. These oral medications prevent cancer cells from being affected by the spike in testosterone production by hampering their ability to absorb the androgen.

LH-RH ANALOGS

LH-RH	Injection route	Injection schedule (months)
Buserelin (Suprefact)	Subcutaneous	1, 2, 3
Goserelin (Zoladex)	Subcutaneous	1, 3
Leuprolide (Lupron)	Intramuscular	1, 3, 4
Leuprolide gel (Eligard)	Subcutaneous	1, 3, 4, 6
Triptorelin pamoate (Trelstar)	Intramuscular	1, 3
Degarelix (Firmagon) (LH-RH antagonist)	Subcutaneous	1

Doctors prescribe anti-androgens for different lengths of time. Some recommend they be taken for one to two months at the beginning of LH-RH analog therapy, while others believe they should be administered continuously in combination with LH-RH analogs to counter the effects of adrenal gland hormones that may remain in the bloodstream. According to the latter group of doctors, this approach (known as maximal androgen blockade) controls the cancer more effectively and improves chances of survival, although the extent to which this is true remains controversial.

A number of years ago, LH-RH antagonists (inhibitors) became available. The results are similar to those obtained with LH-RH analogs but the mechanism of action is different. Unlike LH-RH analogs, LH-RH antagonists do not cause an initial surge in testosterone.

Men who have undergone orchiectomy or who receive LH-RH antagonists do not experience a testosterone surge since they no longer produce the hormone. Anti-androgens are not prescribed for such men, unless the doctor recommends maximal androgen blockade.

Side effects of hormone therapy

Both surgical and medical castration cause a drop in hormone production that inevitably leads to a loss of sex drive. There are

ANTI-ANDROGENS

Anti-androgen	Dose
Bicalutamide (Casodex)	50 mg once daily
Flutamide (Euflex)	50 mg 3 times per day
Cyproterone acetate (Androcur)	100 mg 2 times per day
Nilutamide (Anandron)	150 mg once daily

other side effects as well, including hot flashes, fatigue, anemia, mood swings, a slight increase in mammary gland mass and loss of bone and muscle mass.

Doctors can prescribe medication as needed to reduce the intensity of hot flashes and the extent of bone loss. There is still no standard treatment for the other side effects. While every individual reacts differently to hormonal changes, most men find the side effects fairly tolerable.

Men taking anti-androgen therapy alone (rarely done) will experience a significant increase in mammary gland mass that is more pronounced than that caused by LH-RH analogs or surgical castration. This is the primary side effect of this type of therapy, and patients should be made aware of this.

Long-term complications of hormone therapy
Orchiectomy is, of course, irreversible and the side effects are therefore permanent. Hot flashes and fatigue, however, do tend to ease over time. Bone loss, on the other hand, can lead to osteoporosis. Doctors may prescribe calcium supplements, vitamin D or even medication such as bisphosphonates as preventive measures or treatment (if the bone is significantly weakened by age or by the effects of hormone therapy).

When LH-RH analog therapy is prescribed for a short period, the side effects (those described above) generally disappear soon after treatment ends. However, the longer the therapy lasts, the more likely that the side effects will persist. While a man's breasts stop increasing in size soon after treatment ends, the process cannot be reversed and his breasts will not get smaller again. After two years of continuous therapy, testosterone levels may never return to normal and side effects can become permanent, much as in orchiectomy. Note that a return to normal testosterone levels after a short treatment does not necessarily mean the cancer will recur.

Men taking LH-RH analogs report that the scrotum tends to shrink over the course of treatment. This is because the testicles eventually atrophy if they stop functioning for a significant period of time.

CONTINUOUS OR INTERMITTENT LH-RH ANALOG THERAPY?

In advanced prostate cancer, whatever the form, standard practice was to prescribe LH-RH analog treatment as a lifelong therapy.

Over the last few years, however, "intermittent" therapy has become more popular. This approach involves administering LH-RH analogs for six to eight months until prostate-specific antigen (PSA) levels drop and stabilize, and symptoms disappear. Treatment resumes when PSA levels begin to climb again, which can happen months or sometimes years later. In intermittent therapy, it is recommended that anti-androgens be taken at the beginning of each new treatment cycle.

In theory, intermittent therapy lets the patient reclaim a "normal" sex life and live free of side effects during the time he is not taking medication.

A recent study confirms that intermittent hormone therapy is as effective as continuous hormone therapy in cases of PSA recurrence without the presence of metastases (see "Recurrence after treatment of localized cancer").

Patients should discuss these issues thoroughly with their doctors.

A man's loss of sex drive and his inability to achieve natural erections can have a direct impact on his personal life. If the man has also undergone a radical prostatectomy or radiation therapy, his erectile dysfunction will be even more pronounced. Though they lack the physical desire for sex, some men still try out medical techniques to help them achieve erections (see Chapter 6). However, many eventually come to accept the loss of a full sex life as the price paid for slowing the progression of the disease and increasing their life expectancy.

Medical follow-up of hormone therapy

Every three to six months, the patient meets with his doctor, who performs the occasional DRE and orders regular PSA tests to monitor for increases suggesting the cancer has recurred.

RECURRENCE AFTER TREATMENT OF LOCALIZED CANCER

If cancer returns after radical prostatectomy or radiation therapy—either alone or in combination with hormone therapy—it is considered to be advanced. This is true whether the recurrence is localized or distant. Localized recurrence means cancer cells have escaped the effects of treatment but remain in the same anatomical area as the treated prostate. Distant recurrence means the tumour is located in a part of the body far from the original cancer. Though recurrences can occur at any time, the risk of recurrence after initial treatment diminishes with time. Five years is often quoted as the magic number, but there is no absolute guarantee of remaining cancer-free from that time on. Long-term follow-up is still required.

Recurrence is generally first signalled by an increase in PSA levels. The rate at which PSA level rises (doubling time) and the grade and stage of the original tumour help the doctor determine whether the recurrence is most likely localized or distant. The faster the PSA rises and the higher the grade or stage of the original tumour, the more likely that the recurrence is distant.

Recurrence after radical prostatectomy

In most cases, PSA levels provide an early warning, raising a flag several months or years before a recurrence is widespread enough to cause problems or be detected by radiology or on a physical exam. If begun at a very early stage, hormone therapy significantly impedes the progression of the disease.

In some cases of localized recurrence, it is even possible to completely cure the disease through radiation therapy alone or in combination with hormone therapy.

Patients with slowly progressing recurring cancer, either localized or distant, may be good candidates for intermittent hormone therapy (see box, "Continuous or intermittent LH-RH analog therapy?").

If the recurrence appears to be localized, slow-growing and not particularly worrisome in any other respect, the doctor may recommend that the patient forgo treatment altogether. For example, in a case where PSA levels begin to rise five years after an operation, there will likely be no metastasis for another 10 or 15 years. If the patient is already elderly or has a short life expectancy, it might be better to avoid or delay treatment instead of introducing hormone therapy that will impair his quality of life. If the patient is younger and has a longer life expectancy, the doctor will probably take a more aggressive approach and prescribe radiation therapy, either alone or in combination with hormone therapy.

Once the decision has been made to forgo radiation therapy, the patient can choose to wait for a significant increase in PSA levels before beginning hormone therapy, so as to postpone the side effects described above. Of course, if the progression of the disease becomes worrisome, treatment can begin immediately. Every case is unique, and the patient must weigh the pros and cons carefully in close consultation with his doctor.

Recurrence after radiation therapy (external or brachytherapy)

Hormone therapy is often considered the standard treatment for cancer recurrence after radiation therapy. In the absence of metastasis, intermittent hormone therapy is a valid option (see box, "Continuous or intermittent LH-RH analog therapy?"). Again, if the recurrence is slow-growing, the patient can choose to delay treatment.

In rare cases, radical prostatectomy is recommended, but only if the doctor is convinced that the recurrence is limited to the prostate gland. This approach causes more pronounced side effects than radical prostatectomy as a first-line treatment (see Chapter 4). Furthermore, because radiation therapy burns the tissue, a subsequent radical prostatectomy can cause further damage to the bladder, urethra, rectum and erectile nerves. Sometimes the doctor is forced to abandon the procedure upon discovering the extent of the disease or the state of the tissue after making the skin incision. In such cases, hormone therapy is prescribed instead.

High-intensity focused ultrasound (HIFU) and cryotherapy are new options currently being studied. These options are discussed in Chapter 4. HIFU involves inserting an ultrasound probe that sends intense heat to the prostate in the hope of destroying prostatic tissue and the cancer within. Cryotherapy involves placing the patient under general or epidural anesthesia and inserting probes containing liquid nitrogen through the perineum (the area between the testicles and the rectum) into the prostate to freeze the gland and destroy the cancerous cells. These approaches are only used when the doctor believes the recurrence is limited to the prostate. They can cause side effects, including urinary incontinence, rectal lesions and erectile dysfunction. Since their long-term effectiveness is still unknown, they are offered in only a few Canadian health centres. Other forms of investigational therapy are being tested in the setting of recurrence after radiation therapy so in the future there may be more choices for patients.

LOCALLY ADVANCED NON-METASTATIC CANCER

The treatment of localized prostate cancer (in other words, cancer that has not metastasized) is discussed in Chapter 4. This category includes cancers that have moved beyond the prostate gland itself and are therefore too advanced to benefit from radical prostatectomy or radiation therapy alone.

For example, cancers at stage T3 (the cancer has spread beyond the capsule of the prostate) or T4 (the tumour has reached neighbouring tissue such as the bladder, the external sphincter or the rectum) are not limited to the prostate gland though there are no detectable metastases according to the bone scan and other diagnostic exams.

In these cases, hormone therapy is frequently recommended as a complement to radical prostatectomy or radiation therapy. (Radiation therapy is usually prescribed for stages T3+ and T4, since the cancer is too advanced to be treated surgically.)

Hormone therapy is generally prescribed for two or three years in combination with radiation. A study published in the prestigious New England Journal of Medicine in the late 1990s demonstrated that this approach lowers the risk of the cancer spreading and prolongs survival. However, if the tumour is deemed worrisome enough, the doctor can immediately prescribe hormone therapy for life.

Medical follow-up and regular PSA measurements allow the doctor to judge whether or not the cancer has stabilized. If PSA levels begin to climb again, hormone therapy is resumed, generally for life; if they stay where they are for five years or more, the cancer is possibly cured.

An experimental treatment for locally advanced non-metastasized cancers is currently being studied. This treatment entails combining hormone therapy with chemotherapy (see "Chemotherapy" below) using a drug called docetaxel (Taxotere) plus radiation therapy or radical prostatectomy. It is hoped that this approach will help cure more patients with a high risk of recurrence. If you are found to have a high-risk prostate cancer, you should speak to

METASTATIC CANCER

Nodal metastasis
Metastasis to the lymph nodes can be predicted using risk evaluation tables like the Partin tables (see Chapter 4) or confirmed with a lymphadenectomy (surgical removal of lymph nodes which are then analyzed under a microscope). The standard treatment is lifelong hormone therapy, which could involve orchiectomy. If the patient prefers LH-RH analog therapy (the most common choice), anti-androgen treatment may also be prescribed.

Prostate cancer most commonly spreads to the lymph nodes and the bones. Studies published in the late 1990s show that if hormone therapy is started as soon as nodal metastasis is found instead of waiting for the onset of bone metastasis, the chances of survival are significantly better.

In some cases, however, the doctor may prefer to wait and monitor the patient's PSA levels. In approximately 10 to 15 percent of nodal metastases, PSA levels remain stable for a number of years. With regular follow-up every three to six months, intervention is possible as soon as PSA levels begin to rise, months or even years before the cancer has metastasized anywhere else.

The decision to wait is generally made to avoid side effects of hormone therapy as long as possible.

Bone metastasis
Cancer that has spread to the lymph nodes may eventually attack the bones, particularly the pelvis and spine. When metastases are severe, the following symptoms may eventually appear: pain in the lower back or hips, numbness or paralysis of the lower limbs (metastases in the vertebrae can put pressure on the spinal cord), fatigue, loss of appetite and paleness (due to anemia). Bones also become very fragile and fracture easily.

Hormone therapy is prescribed as soon as the doctor observes the presence of bone metastasis, whether or not the patient is experiencing pain. The treatment is almost always continuous and for life.

Hormone therapy eases the pain and prolongs the patient's life appreciably.

While intermittent hormone therapy (see box, "Continuous or intermittent LH-RH analog therapy?") in cases of bone metastasis has been studied and proved possible in some patients, most experts consider continuous, lifelong hormone therapy to be the best option for patients with metastatic prostate cancer.

Encouraging findings for patients recently diagnosed with metastatic prostate cancer were reported in 2014. After 10 years of research, it was found that patients live much longer and metastasis-related symptoms are delayed if hormone therapy is combined with docetaxel early on (see "Chemotherapy" below) rather than waiting for the cancer to become resistant to hormone therapy.

WHEN HORMONE THERAPY IS NOT ENOUGH

Once hormone therapy (either surgical or medical castration) begins, PSA levels should stabilize or decrease. A continued increase indicates progression despite hormone treatment, and the disease is then referred to as castration-resistant prostate cancer (CRPC). There are two types of CRPC: CRPC with detectable metastasis (or metastatic CRPC) and CRPC without detectable metastasis (or non-metastatic CRPC).

If the patient is also taking anti-androgens and his PSA is still rising, the cancer cells may have mutated and begun using the anti-androgen drug as a stimulant, like testosterone. The first step then is to stop or change the anti-androgen. Between 15 and 30 percent of men will experience a temporary drop in PSA levels when they stop or change anti-androgens. Usually no further treatment will be required until PSA levels begin to rise again. It is important, however, that LH-RH therapy be continued to maintain low testosterone levels.

If circumstances permit, the patient may take part in a clinical trial designed to find better ways of treating this stage of the disease.

Castration-resistant prostate cancer (CRPC) with detectable metastasis

In this type of cancer, diagnostic exams such as bone and CT scans can detect metastasis. Sadly, since curing the disease is no longer possible at this stage, prolonging life and preserving the patient's quality of life become the number-one priority. The doctor attempts to delay complications due to metastasis—pain, bone fractures, loss of mobility, paralysis, etc.—for as long as possible. As soon as the cancer reaches the castration-resistant stage and metastasis is detectable, hormone therapy, is no longer enough on its own.

Chemotherapy

In the early 1990s, it was discovered that chemotherapy (which involves intravenous injections that kill cancer cells) could help ease pain in patients suffering from CRPC with detectable metastasis. At the time, a combination of mitoxantrone (once every three weeks) plus daily prednisone was administered. Because this palliative chemotherapy weakened the heart muscle, the patient could receive no more than 10 or 12 injections. Used alone or in combination with analgesics and/or palliative radiation therapy, chemotherapy improved patients' quality of life, although it did not prolong life.

Docetaxel (Taxotere)

In June 2004, a remarkable development took place. Two international studies confirmed that chemotherapy with docetaxel (Taxotere) relieved symptoms even more effectively than mitoxantrone. In fact, docetaxel not only improved quality of life but also prolonged life by about 25 percent compared to patients at the same disease stage who did not get docetaxel. For the first time, it was shown that a patient suffering from CRPC with detectable metastasis could live longer and better thanks to chemotherapy.

The treatment involves administering docetaxel injections every three weeks. In some cases, the dosage can be reduced and the drug administered once a week to lessen adverse effects on the bone marrow. The treatment takes approximately one half-hour to administer and is given on an out-patient basis at the clinic. The number of chemotherapy cycles (injections) varies according to the patient's tolerance and response. Generally, about six to ten cycles are administered. The way we determine if docetaxel is working is by checking if PSA levels have been affected (they should go down or at least stop increasing as fast as before) and if symptoms due to the disease are improving. Rarely are changes seen on an X-ray, since it is difficult to determine if a treatment is working in the bone. In many patients, improvements in PSA levels and symptoms are seen after as few as two docetaxel treatments. This is extremely encouraging, and often renews hope and gives patients the motivation to continue their fight against the disease.

The mere fact that a patient with CRPC with detectable metastasis can now live longer has forever changed the treatment of this type of disease and opened the door to a new field of research.

Men with metastasis at diagnosis

Docetaxel has recently been used when patients present with metastasis at the time of diagnosis. Fortunately, this occurs infrequently in North America. In such patients, hormone therapy usually works for one or two years before signs of becoming resistant appear. Two studies confirm that docetaxel in combination with hormone therapy at the time of diagnosis results in much longer survival than waiting for patients to be resistant to hormone therapy to start docetaxel.

The patients who benefited the most were those with several sites of metastasis (that is, the cancer had spread to several bones or was attacking vital organs such as the liver or lungs).

Hormone therapy was given in the standard fashion, but docetaxel chemotherapy was added every three weeks for six treatments. This regimen was easier for patients to tolerate, and they also responded far better than when given the standard hormone therapy alone: chances of PSA dropping to zero doubled and patients remained stable for much longer. In addition, older patients (over 70) benefited as much as younger ones. In sum, chemotherapy continues to play an important role in the treatment of prostate cancer that has spread to other organs, and it seems that the earlier it is administered the better.

Research protocols are ongoing to determine the drug's potential in combination with other treatments such as radical prostatectomy or radiation therapy for patients with more aggressive cancers. To improve docetaxel results, scientists are also studying how it combines with other drugs, and so far, a number of important steps have been made in this area. The hope is that research will lead to a longer and better quality of life.

Side effects of docetaxel
Docetaxel does cause certain side effects, the most common being hair loss, nausea, fatigue and lowered white blood cell count (which increases the risk of infection). Most of the time, these effects fade and disappear after the treatment is complete. Despite the side effects, however, docetaxel is generally

well-tolerated, even by the elderly, and improves a patient's quality of life considerably. Another recent discovery is that some patients may benefit from docetaxel more than once. If a patient is in good shape after completing a treatment regimen and the cancer progresses again, it is possible to restart docetaxel and see if the patient benefits again. In a significant proportion of patients, there is the possibility of a second response and new hope.

Treatment options after docetaxel

Cabazitaxel (Jevtana)

Until 2010, there were no options proven effective for patients who had received docetaxel (Taxotere) and continued to deteriorate. Finally, after years of research, cabazitaxel (Jevtana) was demonstrated effective in prolonging life in such patients.

CHEMOTHERAPY (NOT AS BAD AS IT SOUNDS!)

Until recently, there was no form of therapy capable of improving survival in patients with castration-resistant prostate cancer (CRPC). The discovery that docetaxel (Taxotere) can significantly prolong life at this stage while also improving quality of life and controlling pain has profoundly altered the way we treat these patients. It has also led to an explosion of research in the field of advanced prostate cancer and into earlier uses of chemotherapy in high-risk patients with localized prostate cancer. In patients who do not respond to docetaxel or who eventually recur, there is now hope with a new chemotherapy called cabazitaxel (Jevtana) that may further prolong life.

Like docetaxel, this chemotherapy is given every three weeks by injection. Well-tolerated, cabazitaxel was found to prolong life by 30 percent in patients who recurred after receiving docetaxel. This is an extraordinary finding that has given hope to patients with no other options. Cabazitaxel was the first drug to be approved in North America for second-line therapy after docetaxel. Side effects are quite well-tolerated, with diarrhea and low white blood cells being the most frequent side effects.

New generation hormone therapy

Around 2011, a striking discovery was made: new forms of hormone therapy were found to be effective in patients thought to be refractory to hormones. This discovery came after many years of research which confirmed that prostate cancer progressing on hormone therapy is very dependent on the minute amount of male hormones still in circulation. The older hormone therapies are still useful and must continue to be used, but adding a new generation of hormonal agents, such as abiraterone and enzalutamide, offers substantial benefits for patients.

Abiraterone (Zytiga)

Abiraterone (Zytiga) is an oral medication that inhibits the production of almost all hormones that can stimulate cancer cells—those produced by the adrenal glands as well as those produced by the cancer cells themselves, even in castrated patients. In a large study in 2011 of patients with castration-resistant prostate cancer (CRPC) with detectable metastasis (see above) who progressed after receiving docetaxel, abiraterone was found to improve survival by about 35 percent in patients who received it compared to those who did not. More recently, abiraterone was shown to be effective in delaying cancer progression and prolonging life in patients who had not yet received chemotherapy (see "Chemotherapy" above). Patients on abiraterone must take a small dose of cortisone daily to reduce the risk of side effects and help decrease disease symptoms. Although serious side effects are infrequent, some patients may develop swelling of the legs, fatigue or hypertension when taking this medication, and regular blood tests as well as checkups are required. Importantly, abiraterone has been shown to significanly improve quality of life and prolong survival. This class of medication is often used first when patients are diagnosed with metastatic CRPC. Unfortunately the cancer will often develop resistance to this and every drug we use. When this happens with abiraterone, patients will often be treated with chemotherapy (see above) or radium-223 (see below).

Enzalutamide (Xtandi)

In January 2012, a new drug, enzalutamide (Xtandi), demonstrated very encouraging efficacy in patients with metastatic CRPC that recurred after chemotherapy. This oral medication targets the androgen receptor and blocks the effect of any circulating androgens. In many patients, the cancer regresses when these receptors are blocked. Patients who received this treatment during the study survived about 35 percent longer than those who did not. Like abiraterone, enzalutamide was also studied in patients who had not yet received chemotherapy: study results showed patients who received enzalutamide lived longer, and their cancers remained stable for much longer, than those who did not. Although serious side effects are infrequent, patients on enzalutamide may develop fatigue or hypertension. There is also a very low risk of seizure. Regular blood tests and checkups are required. Enzalutamide has been shown to significantly improve quality of life and prolong survival. Like abiraterone, this class of medication is an option that can be used when patients are initially diagnosed with metastatic CRPC. When patients develop resistance they will often be treated with chemotherapy (see above) or radium-223 (see below).

Managing bone metastases

Radium-223 (Xofigo)

The most recent agent shown to be effective in metastatic CRPC is a radioactive agent called radium-223 (Xofigo). This agent targets bone metastases in patients who have failed or were unable to receive chemotherapy. A 30-percent improvement in survival has been demonstrated in patients taking this agent.

Radium-223 is a radioactive liquid given as an injection into a vein. The injection takes only one to two minutes and is given every four weeks in a dedicated treatment room. A maximum of six treatments are given. The body treats radium-223 like calcium. From your bloodstream, it is taken directly into the bones, especially where there are bone metastases, detected in advance by a bone scan.

The treatment does not require hospitalization. Radium-223 poses no exposure hazard to the patient's family or the general public once administered as long as the simple recommendations given by the doctor administering the treatment are followed.

Side effects of radium-223

Side effects of radium-223 are generally very mild and temporary and can include nausea, diarrhea and vomiting (rare). Radium-223 can also cause blood cell counts to drop, increasing the risks of bleeding, infection and anemia. The side effects diminish with time and tend to disappear have all treatments have ended.

Results and medical monitoring with radium-223

Radium-223 prolongs survival and significantly improves quality of life in most patients by reducing bone pain. In the days prior to administration of the treatment, blood is drawn so that blood counts, renal function and bone remodeling associated with active metasases can be monitored. Radium-223 has no significant impact on PSA levels, which may continue to rise even though the treatment is effective. PSA is thus not necessarily measured during the treatment.

Bone-targeted supportive therapy
In 2002, bisphosphonates were approved as a treatment to alleviate bone pain and stabilize bones weakened by cancer. So far, the only bisphosphonate with proven effectiveness is zoledronic acid (Zometa), administered once every four weeks in the clinic. Bisphosphonates can stop or slow the progression of bone destruction due to metastasis, thereby reducing the risk of fracture. When used in patients with CRPC and bone metastases, bisphosphonates can reduce the risk of complications due to metastasis and lessen the need for painkillers and palliative radiation therapy.

In 2010, a new class of bone-targeted therapy was found to be effective for the prevention of bone complications due to metastasis. This new class of drugs blocks something called RANK ligand, which plays a central role in bone destruction in the presence of metastasis. Denosumab (Xgeva) is the first agent in this class of drugs demonstrated to be effective and has, in fact, proved slightly more effective than zoledronic acid in reducing bone complications in men with metastatic CRPC. Denosumab is given every four weeks in the clinic. Denosumab is called Prolia when it is taken every six months at a lower dose. Prolia has also been demonstrated very effective in reducing bone loss (preventing osteoporosis) due to medical castration (see above) and in lowering the associated risk of fractures.

Palliative radiation therapy destroys metastatic cells in the bone that cause pain (in the spine, hips and back, for example). This does not change the course of the disease, but it can provide rapid relief of pain and strengthen the bone, thereby reducing the risk of fractures. In most cases, palliative radiation therapy is used when pain-relieving drugs are insufficient or the risk of fracture is high. However, because any area of the body can generally be irradiated only once, palliative radiation therapy is usually a last resort. If the pain returns to the irradiated area, only painkillers and bone-targeted therapy can help. These medications can also be used in combination with palliative radiation therapy.

Castration-resistant prostate cancer (CRPC) without detectable metastasis

This is a situation in which PSA continues to rise even though the patient is taking hormone therapy. It is called castration-resistant prostate cancer (CRPC) without detectable metastasis or non-metastatic castration-resistant prostate cancer (nmCRPC) because metastases are not yet perceptible through bone or CT-scan, though it is likely to have started on a microscopic level and to eventually be visible and cause the patient symptoms.

Until recently, there was no treatment proven to help in such situations, and doctors were advised to perform regular follow-ups every three or six months until metastasis was confirmed. Only then would treatment be available.

Non-metastatic CRPC has been the most studied area in prostate cancer research in recent years, with the goal to find medications that can prevent or delay the onset of metastasis.

In 2018, positive results were reported with two agents, both demonstrated to delay the onset of metastasis by approximately two years in patients with rapidly rising PSA levels (high-risk non-metastatic CRPC). Enzalutamide, already used in metastatic CRPC, caused a very significant delay in metastasis in the target patients. Apalutamide, a new drug very similar to enzalutamide, showed similar results. It is very exciting to finally have something effective to offer patients at high risk of becoming metastatic. It is still too early to know if patients will live longer with these drugs. In addition, since prostate cancer evolves differently, not all patients will need these preventive drugs. Fortunately, there are ways to help doctors and patients make the decision that is most appropriate in each particular case.

SUMMARY

It is extremely encouraging that in less than 15 years five new drugs have become available, in addition to docetaxel (Taxotere), for patients with CRPC, with or without metastasis, who previously had run out of options. Many patients now have access to more than one new drug that can prolong survival and improve quality of life. Although these are important findings, intense research continues, since patients unfortunately cannot be cured at this stage of the disease.

CHAPTER 5 – TREATMENT OF ADVANCED PROSTATE CANCER

ONE PERSON'S STORY

Name: Robert	**Age:** 67 years old
Occupation: Volunteer chauffeur	

Robert was diagnosed with prostate cancer three years ago. At that time, the cancer had spread to his bones. He was prescribed an LH-RH analog (hormone therapy) and did well until a few months ago, with his PSA dropping from 150 at the time of diagnosis to 1. Six months ago, his PSA began to rise, and he developed intense pain in his hip and lower spine. He received radiation therapy and zoledronic acid, and these relieved most of the pain in his hip. He then began chemotherapy with docetaxel (Taxotere) every three weeks at the outpatient oncology clinic. His PSA dropped from 50 to 2.5, he felt much better and his pain disappeared completely. Apart from hair loss, he tolerated the chemotherapy quite well. It has now been three months since he finished his chemotherapy, and he complains of some recurrence of pain in his lower back. In addition, his PSA has gone up to 30. Otherwise, he is feeling very well.

His options were discussed with him. Since he is feeling healthy and had a good experience with previous chemotherapy, he has decided to begin cabazitaxel (Jevtana), to be administered every three weeks. He remains optimistic, continues to eat as well as possible and stays active. He is well aware that a cure is not possible, but he is encouraged by the positive results reported with cabazitaxel, abiraterone, enzalutamide and radium-223. These options are likely to help when the time comes for more treatment. He knows that abiraterone is another option if needed in the future, as is MDV3100. He is also aware that he could have access to new therapies by participating in ongoing clinical research. Given the new therapies available, he is optimistically looking forward to being present for his grandson's birth in six months.

CHAPTER 6
LIVING WITH PROSTATE CANCER

Few things are as difficult as learning that you have cancer. The word itself casts a chilling shadow, as does the knowledge of the side effects and complications from treatment. The person hearing this terrifying news knows that life will never be the same, and emotions can range from denial to anger, despair to hope, and courage to fear, for both the patient and his or her loved ones. All of this is completely normal.

Much like the impact of breast cancer, the psychological effects of prostate cancer are deeply troubling to the sufferer. Prostate cancer touches a very sensitive place in the male psyche. For one thing, a man's physical integrity is threatened by the risk of erectile dysfunction and urinary incontinence brought about by treatment. But even more profoundly, the disease troubles a man's very perception of himself, his body, his sexuality and his intimate relationships.

To be sure, a man of 82 who develops prostate cancer does not go through the same thing as a man of 49 who is still sexually virile and able to reproduce. Not only does the latter fear dying young, he also worries about losing his sexual powers. He might feel that "it's all over," that he is "no longer a man" and that his partner will abandon him. Most men in this age bracket are ready to do anything to cure the disease and will undergo the most aggressive treatment available.

Older men tend to react differently. Generally less sexually active, these men may find it a little easier to accept having their prostate removed or losing the ability to achieve erections. On the other hand, they may have more trouble dealing with treatment side effects like urinary incontinence and be less willing to spend a great deal of time in hospital. They might therefore choose to undergo treatments with "milder" side effects.

SUPPORT FROM THE DOCTOR

A patient with prostate cancer needs psychological support throughout his illness. The primary person to provide this support is the patient's urologist, who will follow him for years—assisted by a radiation oncologist if the patient needs radiation therapy and a hematologist-oncologist if chemotherapy is required. The urologist's attitude will have a strong influence on the patient's outlook during treatment.

Professional ethics prohibit a doctor from concealing the diagnosis from the patient as well as from revealing it to the patient's loved ones without the patient's prior knowledge. The patient has a right to know the state of his health and needs this information in order to make informed choices. The only situations in which a doctor is permitted to conceal the diagnosis are when the patient is suffering from major depression, has a psychotic disorder or a history of suicidal behaviour, or does not have the mental capacity to understand the doctor's explanations.

When the doctor shares the diagnosis with the patient, a space is created in which the two can nurture an open and frank relationship. The doctor must first respond to the patient's fears about operations, radiation therapy, losing his sexual capacity and dying. He or she must play down the drama of the situation, as long as this does not bend the truth.

It is very rare for a patient to want to hear all the details on the first visit. Once the word "cancer" is uttered, a mental barrier goes up and the patient will likely not absorb some of the information that follows. Not surprisingly, the patient needs a little time. The doctor must be empathetic, know how to provide information in small, digestible portions and be able to anticipate the most important questions.

The doctor should conclude every visit by asking the patient what he remembers from the meeting, in order to correct any misapprehensions or fill in any gaps. It is also up to the patient to ask for clarifications; the patient should never leave the doctor's office without answers or without understanding what was discussed. Some patients bring loved ones to the consultation for comfort and support during this process, and these people can also help clarify a point if the patient is unsure.

IT'S STILL POSSIBLE TO START A FAMILY

Some younger men fear they will no longer be able to have children after being treated for prostate cancer. Certainly, there is reason for concern. For example, ejaculation is impossible after radical prostatectomy and not very likely after radiation therapy. Hormone therapy creates a different kind of problem by wiping out a man's sex drive.

However, a man who would still like to start a family can have his sperm frozen before treatment begins. Later on, whenever the couple chooses, doctors can artificially inseminate the man's partner. This technique is usually successful.

The patient must take an active part in the choice of treatment. The doctor carefully explains all therapeutic options, detailing their benefits, side effects and long-term consequences. The patient can then weigh the pros and cons of each option and make an informed choice. While it is usually a good idea for the patient's partner or other loved one to take part in the consultation, the patient should not be influenced by the opinions of others. The patient alone must make the decision, because he alone will undergo the treatment and live with its outcome.

If the patient does not get along well with his doctor, he has the right to choose another. This is not a huge problem and will have no negative effect on treatment.

MEDICAL FOLLOW-UP

The patient is followed for a minimum of five years, no matter how advanced the prostate cancer when it is detected. Digital rectal exams and prostate-specific antigen (PSA) tests are performed regularly to follow the progression of the disease. PSA levels should diminish and stabilize after treatment, so an increase generally indicates a recurrence.

More and more cancer-treating hospitals are adopting a broad, multidisciplinary approach to the disease. This means that in addition to providing medical care, they promote a more global vision of the patient that recognizes the person's psychological, social, spiritual and religious qualities. By providing information, professional support services and personalized follow-up that meets the individual patient's needs, these hospitals make it a little easier to live with the illness.

WHO DOES WHAT?

When a patient and his family are experiencing distress or difficulties, there are a number of people in the hospital setting who can help. Who to turn to depends first and foremost on the nature of the problem, but also on the patient's preferences. To make an informed decision, the patient should discuss the matter with the attending physician or any other member of the healthcare team involved in his medical follow-up. The patient can obtain help from several sources at once, or first from one and then another professional.

- **The psychiatrist** is a medical specialist who can diagnose psychosocial problems, evaluate underlying physical disorders and prescribe medication. The psychiatrist can also treat patients for pain. A psychiatrist can help the patient physically as well as psychologically.

- **The psychologist** can help in coping with emotional or psychological reactions to the disease and its treatment. He or she can also help in understanding the reactions of family members. The goal of consulting a psychologist is to improve quality of life, psychological health and the patient's and the family's coping capabilities.

- **A sex therapist** can help the patient and his partner adapt their sexuality to the changes that take place after treatment.

- The role of the **social worker** is to promote the social functioning of the patient. The social worker works with the patient and his family. He or she may also assist the patient with procedures for obtaining financial assistance required during cancer treatments. The social worker also works with the healthcare team to organize the patient's discharge from the hospital with the help of resources in the community (CLSC, rehabilitation centres, etc.)

- **The spiritual advisor** offers religious and spiritual support to people who are hospitalized and their loved ones.

SEX

For many men, the most difficult part is the impact of treatment on their sex life, as their emotional life is affected. Prostate cancer treatments can affect erectile function. With erectile-nerve sparing, about 50 percent of men who undergo a radical prostatectomy (complete removal of the prostate) will develop permanent erectile dysfunction. When the surgeon is unable to spare the erectile nerves, erectile dysfunction is permanent in virtually all patients. The disorder occurs immediately, but erectile function gradually improves over the first two years after surgery. After external-beam radiation therapy, 40 to 60 percent of men will develop permanent erectile disorders. Permanent erectile dysfunction is less common after brachytherapy, but still affects 20 to 50 percent of men treated (see Chapter 4). Hormone therapy causes erectile dysfunction indirectly, because the suppression of androgens wipes out a man's sex drive.

Treatments also affect ejaculation. After a radical prostatectomy, a man is permanently unable to ejaculate, as the surgeon has removed the prostate and the seminal vesicles and has severed the vas deferens. Radiation therapy (either external or brachytherapy) significantly reduces the amount of ejaculate and makes it next to impossible for the man to procreate.

On the other hand, a man's libido remains intact after surgery, external radiation therapy or brachytherapy, and orgasm is still possible. Most patients eventually recover the ability to achieve erection (naturally or with the help of treatment) and are able to lead satisfying sex lives.

Things are a little different for men who undergo hormone therapy, which blocks production of testosterone and causes loss of libido. A man thus loses all interest in sex. If the hormone therapy lasts for under a year, the man will very likely regain his sexual desire once the treatment ends. However, the longer the hormone therapy lasts, the higher the risk of permanent libido loss.

Oral treatments for erectile dysfunction

Viagra (sildenafil), Cialis (tadalafil) and Levitra (vardenafil hydrochloride) are the treatments of choice for erectile dysfunction. With the same mechanisms of action and comparable side effects (the most common being headache, sudden facial redness and digestive problems), these medications are all very similar. Their durations of action differ, however: four to eight hours for Viagra and Levitra; and 24 hours for Cialis. All three drugs can be taken as needed 30 to 60 minutes before initiating sexual activity. A low dose of Cialis can also be taken on a daily basis to improve erection spontaneity. Deciding which of these drugs to take is a personal matter, as some men tolerate one better than the others, or get better results with one of the three. The doctor's job is to help the patient determine which product is most suitable for him and to ensure there are no contraindications: these drugs may not be taken by patients who take nitroglycerin for angina pectoris, have severe high blood pressure, experience chest pain during sexual intercourse or have recently had a stroke or a heart attack (infarct).

These medications for erectile dysfunction do not act on the brain or provoke automatic erections; they simply give a little "boost" to the normal erection process. Upon sexual stimulation, erectile nerves emit chemical substances (neurotransmitters) that bring about a dilation of the blood vessels in the penis, resulting in engorgement of the penile tissues and erection. However, after treatment for prostate cancer, the erectile nerves may have some trouble doing their job properly. Viagra, Cialis or Levitra can make it easier to maintain an erection because they help prevent the natural breakdown of neurotransmitters.

The duration of action varies according to the product, but all make it possible for a man to achieve erection in about 30 minutes. However, these drugs are not aphrodisiacs, and the man must be sexually stimulated for them to work. In addition, they are not magic potions: they cannot iron out relationship problems or kindle desire. Some men with prostate cancer feel they are no longer desirable, for example, particularly if they suffer from low self-esteem or their partner is not supportive. This can cause a loss of sexual desire, and pills will not be much help.

Loss of sex drive can also be due to performance anxiety, the man being so intensely concerned with his sexual performance that he loses his ability to perform. Other possible culprits include alcohol, depression or hormone therapy. The latter alters the male sex drive in such a way that pills will likely have very little effect.

Viagra, Cialis and Levitra are about 50 percent effective in men who have had radical prostatectomy, depending on the degree to which the doctor was able to spare the nerves during surgery. If the nerves are very damaged, these medications will probably have little effect. Similarly, the drugs have about a 50 percent success rate in men who have undergone radiation therapy (external or brachytherapy), since such therapy can also damage the nerves. If the patient does not get the hoped-for results, the doctor may suggest other solutions. Whatever the treatment, however, it is likely that the patient will be required to follow it for the rest of his life.

Other solutions

If Viagra, Cialis or Levitra do not work, the doctor can recommend the urethral suppository known as MUSE, intracavernous injections, a vacuum pump or, if all else fails, penile implants. There are also "alternative" solutions.

Urethral suppository (or MUSE)

MUSE (Medicated Urethral System of Erection) is a mini-suppository (about the size of a grain of rice) that contains a drug called alprostadil. The suppository is inserted in the urethra (the opening at the top of the penis), and the penis is massaged lightly where the suppository is located to speed up absorption of the drug and increase its effectiveness. The drug causes the blood vessels to expand, and the penis becomes engorged with blood and hardens. Erection occurs automatically in no more than 15 or 20 minutes and generally lasts about one hour, whether or not the man ejaculates. During this time, the penis will remain erect even if sexual relations come to an end. Some patients who have not been successful with oral medications can achieve erection with MUSE.

Urethral suppository (or MUSE*)

Either sitting or standing, gently extend the penis upwards as far as possible, exerting light pressure from the tip to the base. This will straighten and open the urethra.

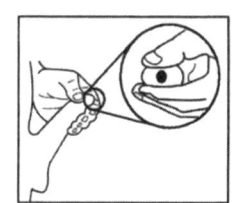

Slowly insert the applicator into the urethra. Be sure to insert the applicator as far as the projecting rim, in order to ensure absorption of the medicated pellet.

Hold the penis in an upward position, extending it as far as possible. Firmly roll the penis between the hands for at least 10 seconds to ensure that the medication is distributed along the walls of the urethra.

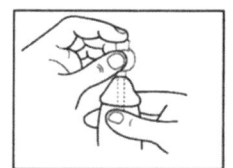

Get up and walk around for 10 minutes while the erection appears. Physical activity increases blood flow to the penis and improves the quality of the erection. Wait at least 10 minutes more before beginning sexual relations.

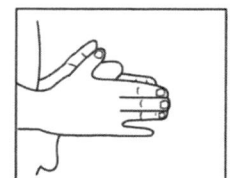

* MUSE is a registered trademark of Vivus Pharmaceuticals.

Intracavernous injection

Intracavernous injection involves injecting a drug or a combination of drugs (alprostadil, papaverine or phentolamine) directly into the corpus cavernosum through the side of the penis. The drugs cause the blood vessels to relax and the penis to engorge with blood. Even without sexual stimulation, the penis can become completely erect in less than

15 minutes and stay that way for an average of 30 minutes to an hour. This treatment is effective in 85 to 90 percent of cases, whatever the origin of the erectile dysfunction. However, while this technique is more effective than MUSE or oral medications, most men do not feel comfortable with penile injections and would prefer to take a pill, if possible.

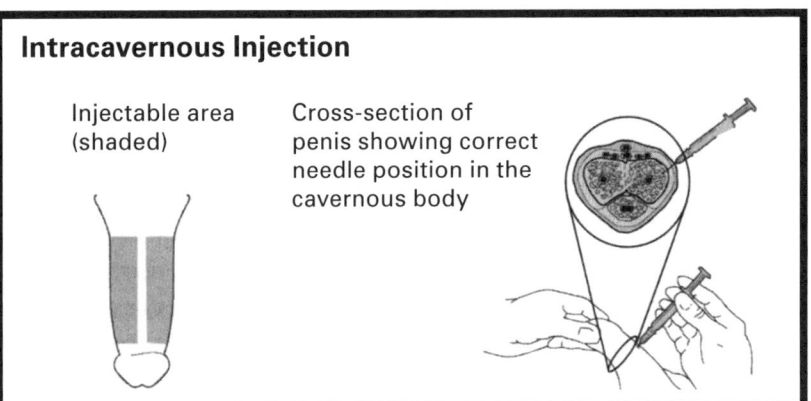

Intracavernous Injection

Injectable area (shaded)

Cross-section of penis showing correct needle position in the cavernous body

Vacuum pump (or external pump)

The vacuum pump is a cylinder open at one end and connected by a tube to a pump that sucks out air. The penis is inserted into the hermetically sealed cylinder and the vacuum created by the pump draws blood into the organ. A safety valve allows the man to control the pressure to avoid damaging tissue. This device can create an automatic erection within a few minutes, which is then sustained by placing an elastic ring around the base of the penis. This compression ring must be removed after 30 to 45 minutes; otherwise, the cells in the penis will be starved of oxygen and blood clots can form in the tissue of the penis. Men who have mastered this technique estimate that it is effective approximately 80 percent of the time.

Vacuum Pump (or external pump)

After the penis is inserted into the cylinder, the pump creates a vacuum drawing blood into the penis.

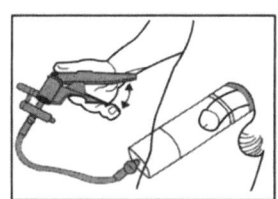

Within minutes, the vacuum causes an erection.

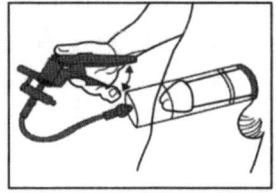

Slide the ring sealing the cylinder to the base of the penis, and withdraw the cylinder.

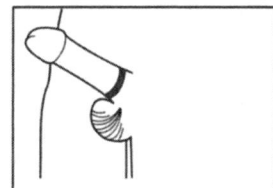

Once the ring is removed from the penis, the organ will return to its normal flaccid state.

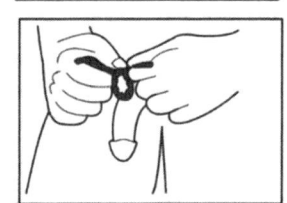

Penile implants

Penile implants are internal prostheses (synthetic cylinders) that are surgically inserted into the cavernous body of the penis. There are two types: semi-rigid (or malleable) or inflatable. The semi-rigid model keeps the penis always at the ready, that is, in a permanent state of semi-erection hard enough for penetration. There is a drawback, since the semi-erect penis can be difficult to camouflage under clothing even though the cylinders of the prosthesis are quite malleable.

Inflatable implants, on the other hand, consist of two cylinders, a reservoir full of saline water (which plays the role of the blood) and a hydraulic pump. The cylinders are inserted into the penis and the reservoir is surgically implanted in the abdomen. These components are linked to a pump that has been surgically inserted into the scrotum. When the pump is activated manually, the saline water enters the cylinders, causing the penis to swell. When sexual relations are over, the pump valve must be pressed again to send the liquid back to the reservoir. These days, this type of implant is considered a last resort and is only recommended if all other methods have failed.

A SEX THERAPIST CAN OFTEN BE HELPFUL

A sex therapist can help the patient and the couple overcome physical problems or learn how to live with them.

For example, the sex therapist provides guidance if the man is unable to achieve erections naturally and the couple is learning how to integrate a medical treatment (oral medication, MUSE or any other type of treatment) into their sex life. The therapist also helps the couple explore other facets of their sexuality and new ways of expressing their love for each other. Sexuality can take a number of forms and still be fulfilling for both partners, as long as it remains a way for the couple to communicate and express their shared happiness.

If the man is undergoing hormone therapy and has therefore lost his sex drive, the sex therapist helps the patient and the couple deal with the situation to prevent suffering, depression and guilt.

Alternative solutions
Some men prefer more "natural" methods. Certain products are reputed to help men achieve erection, such as androstanedione, dehydroepiandrosterone (known as DHEA), ginkgo biloba, yohimbine, ginseng, Avena sativa, Tribulus terrestris, Turnera diffusa and L-arganine. Scientific studies of these substances are few and far between and their effectiveness has not been proven. At the moment, only L-arganine (an essential amino acid) appears to be at all promising and some research is underway. As for the others, no compelling data exists.

SUPPORT FROM THE FAMILY

Cancer upsets and disrupts the entire family. In fact, it's only normal for the patient himself and those close to him to feel different emotions, including fear, sadness and anger. In addition, the patient and those close to him may not experience the same emotions at the same time, complicating communication between them and contributing to everyone's distress. If necessary, family members can speak to professionals, community organizations or support groups for advice (see Useful addresses). It is crucial that the family present a united front and unwavering support for the ill loved one.

To cope with the disease, a man needs the support of his family and the other significant people in his life. Their help—emotional support as well as assistance with practical matters—is crucial. Sometimes all that is required is a friendly presence, an attentive ear, a willingness to do small services—so the patient knows he is not alone. We must never forget that the man with prostate cancer is above all a husband, a father, a brother, a son, a friend ... not just a cancer patient.

The patient must also make an effort to open up to his family and share his fears. This will make him feel better and help him come to terms with his emotions and handle them better. It also makes the patient's loved ones feel more comfortable expressing their own concerns and offering help. The comfort a family can provide is invaluable. This said, the patient must also be allowed to set limits on what he chooses to communicate. An introverted man may have more difficulty sharing his moods, and his family must understand and respect this.

A diagnosis of cancer and its medical management often have a significant impact on a couple. Clearly, the impact of cancer treatment on sexual intimacy is a major preoccupation. The man suffering from erectile dysfunction or loss of sexual desire may fear that his relationship will fall apart and he will lose his life partner. Or, if he is very sick and must spend a great deal of time in the hospital, his partner may be forced to work more to make up for lost income. Such changes happen quickly and can be profoundly disruptive. If there are conflicts or dissatisfaction within the couple, consultation with a psychosocial professional would undoubtedly be helpful.

However, while cancer can be destabilizing, it rarely destroys a couple whose relationship is strong. The partners will stay in touch with their love for one other and, if necessary, will find new ways of expressing tenderness and sexuality.

BEING ILL SHOULDN'T MEAN GIVING UP

Far too often, patients are told they just have to accept the fact that they are sick. In fact, it doesn't have to be that way. While the patient should acknowledge the presence of the cancer, the need for treatment and the consequent side effects, he need not passively accept losing control over his life and resign himself to it.

Adopting a combative attitude and refusing to give up can actually be very good for morale. It may also be the best way to deal with those really tough days.

In older couples, the impact of the disease is felt more in terms of complications from treatment (such as urinary incontinence) and the fact that aging makes frequent trips to the doctor's office more difficult. The patient's spouse and family network may find this demanding, and they should not hesitate to ask the healthcare team for support.

PROFESSIONAL PSYCHOSOCIAL SUPPORT

The patient's healthcare team (including nurses, radiation oncology technologists and volunteers) can offer comfort and support as well as the doctor. Most of the time, the patient's anxiety abates as treatment progresses and he begins to learn what to expect.

In some cases, however, men have difficulty coping with the disease and the treatments. They become withdrawn, isolated and discouraged. Some become depressed or very anxious and may even turn to alcohol. Others have trouble sleeping or concentrating and lose interest in activities they used to enjoy.

A few actually go as far as suicide, although this is extremely rare. Family and friends should keep an eye out for unusual behaviour and speak to the doctor or request guidance from a specialist if anything seems amiss. The doctor can also advise the patient to consult a specialist if a particular kind of support seems required. If the patient himself feels the need, he should never hesitate to consult a professional.

In fact, approximately 40 to 50 percent of men with prostate cancer require some type of psychosocial intervention at some point during their illness. For instance, some men feel particularly anxious after they complete treatment. This can occur even if the patient had no trouble adjusting to the treatment itself, has had regular and reassuring meetings with his doctor and has regained control of his life. Being told that the cancer is in remission and that he does not need to see his doctor for some time can cause anxiety to surface, most likely because the patient fears the disease will reappear now that he is no longer under close medical supervision. Men in situations such as these frequently seek support from a professional.

Even when the disease goes into remission after treatment, the cancer may recur (reappear) or metastasize, and chronic effects may develop—including pain, sexual dysfunction or urinary disorders. When this happens, patients generally need support, from family and friends as well as professionals, to help them cope with the new reality they face.

Sometimes, the cancer cannot be cured. The disease may progress slowly or rapidly, but eventually the patient ends up in palliative care. Most people have difficulty accepting that their life has come to an end and they are about to die. They may feel disappointment, anger, sadness or fear. If the patient's distress is overwhelming, he and his family should seek professional support, from a psychologist or a psychiatrist, for example. A spiritual advisor can also offer comfort. Not all patients in palliative care need this type of support. Some eventually make peace with the inevitable and face this new stage in their life with serenity.

OVERCOMING SHYNESS AND PRIDE

It is well-known that men are less likely than women to consult a professional for psychological problems. Men are generally less willing to open up and some even believe that it is not "manly" to share their most intimate feelings with a professional. Unfortunately, this attitude does not usually change with age.

Not all men with prostate cancer need professional psychosocial support. Indeed, about 55 to 60 percent of patients never consult. However, those who do feel the need for such support should not let their shyness or pride stop them from picking up the phone and making an appointment. It could make a huge difference in their quality of life, both during and after treatment.

To promote psychological well-being, it is important for cancer patients to maintain their physical, social and recreational activities as much as possible. The pleasure these provide helps combat discouragement, pessimism and anxiety. When the disease or its treatment limit what the patient can do, it is important to find ways to ensure the patient can still engage in enjoyable activities and maintain satisfying social contacts.

OTHER SOURCES OF SUPPORT

In addition to the doctor, healthcare team, family, psychiatrist, psychologist, social worker and spiritual advisor, a number of other sources exist to help patients and their families get through the ordeal of prostate cancer.

Local and national organizations provide advice on coping with the disease and its treatment. Some also offer psychological support, home care and travel assistance.

Local support groups are composed of cancer sufferers and survivors. For many, talking about the disease with other men who have had similar experiences is a great source of comfort, understanding and encouragement.

The doctor and the other members of the healthcare team can provide a list of local and national organizations and support groups.

CHAPTER 7
NUTRITIONAL GUIDE

Prostate cancer continues to be an important public health problem in Canada. It is the most commonly diagnosed cancer among men and the third leading cause of cancer-related death among Canadian men. The average risk for a Canadian male of being diagnosed with prostate cancer in his lifetime is approximately one in seven. Although the causes of this common condition remain elusive, we are beginning to learn more and more about the important role that diet plays in the development or progression of early prostate cancer. It is now believed that alterations in diet, coupled with the consumption of certain micronutrients, may have an impact on prostate cancer. This chapter reviews some of the descriptive epidemiology of prostate cancer that leads to belief in the importance of diet. It also outlines a variety of dietary strategies which, alone or in combination, can reduce the risk of prostate cancer or delay the progression of the disease in men who have it.

EPIDEMIOLOGY OF PROSTATE CANCER

Four characteristics of prostate cancer suggest that the environment and dietary factors play an important role in the development and/or progression of the disease. The first is the tremendous variation in prostate cancer incidence and mortality worldwide. In some parts of the world, prostate cancer is a rare occurrence and the risk of dying from the disease quite small. This is particularly true in the Far East, in countries such as China and Japan. On the other hand, prostate cancer statistics in the Western world, particularly in northern Europe and North America, show prostate cancer to be an increasingly common disease.

The second interesting fact about prostate cancer is that men who emigrate from areas of low risk to areas of high risk tend to acquire the risk level of their adopted country. For example, the risk of dying from the disease for the average man in Japan is one-eighth that of the average North American. When this Japanese man moves to the United States, however, his risk of dying from prostate cancer increases to one-half of the American man's. The increase in risk seems to occur after nine to twelve years of residence in the new country. This is extremely important, because if the protection enjoyed by men in China and Japan were due to genetic factors, then it should remain when they move across the globe. If environmental or dietary factors are at the root of the protection, however, then the observed change in mortality rate makes sense. Essentially, it tells us that there is nothing innately different about men in China or Japan with respect to prostate cancer, and that it is probably something in their environment or diet that explains the lower incidence and mortality rates.

The third interesting feature of prostate cancer is that it exists in essentially two forms. The first, known as "latent" or "autopsy" cancers, refers to tiny bits of prostate cancer that develop in men as they age. It can almost be considered a natural part of the aging process, like grey hair and wrinkles. Examination of the prostates of men who die from other causes reveals that at least 80 percent of men in their eighties harbour microscopic prostate cancers. Interestingly, this occurs even in countries where prostate cancer incidence and death rates are low, such as China and Japan. The other form is clinical prostate cancer, which is diagnosed and can be life-threatening. As mentioned, this type of cancer is extremely rare in Japan and China but common in North America. A comparison of clinical prostate cancer and "latent" or "autopsy" cancers reveals that the major difference is in the amount of disease and the fact that in the former, multiple sites in the prostate are affected. There is also a tendency for faster-growing types of cancer in men who have the clinical form of the disease. On the basis of these observations, current thinking is that an environmental factor, such as diet, is probably responsible for converting the small bits of prostate cancer into clinical cancer in unfavourable environments like North America.

    The fourth interesting clinical feature is that prostate cancer actually strikes men in their third decade of life. Detailed autopsy studies of prostates in young trauma victims have shown that one out of every three men in their thirties harbours microscopic prostate cancer. Thus, while prostate cancer tends to appear as a disease in men in their fifties, sixties and seventies, it has actually been present for quite some time. What is particularly interesting here is that if the progress of the smaller tumours present in men in their thirties can be slowed, they may never become larger and more clinically significant as these men age. The men might then die of other natural causes, never knowing that they had small amounts of prostate cancer, much as occurs in Asia now. What is more, given the long timeline due to the disease's slow progression, slowing it down even slightly could have a dramatic impact.

    It is therefore hoped that by altering diet either early or later in life, or by adding certain micronutrient combinations, the growth of pre-existing cancer cells in young men can be slowed to the point that the men will never know they had the disease. This same strategy could also be used in men with later-stage prostate cancers in the event that a few cancer cells survive surgery or radiation treatment.

DIETARY FAT

There is a consistent relationship between the intake of dietary fat and the development of prostate cancer. Men in East Asia are not large consumers of dietary fat. There are four major theories associating dietary fat consumption and prostate cancer. According to the first theory, consumers of large amounts of dietary fat tend to produce larger quantities of male hormones such as testosterone. This has been demonstrated in numerous studies, including studies of identical twins and prison inmates. Because the prostate is a male reproductive gland, it is sensitive to male androgens and therefore larger amounts of androgen may put men at a higher risk of prostate cancer.

According to the second theory, it is not dietary fat per se that is responsible for prostate cancer, but rather environmental contaminants (such as pesticides) that become dissolved in dietary fat and are passed up the food chain. Indeed, some pesticides do have testosterone-like properties. If this is the case, then fat itself is not harmful; it is simply a carrier for other harmful substances.

The third major theory posits that certain fatty acids may be responsible. In a variety of studies, fatty acids (linoleic acid, among others) have been associated with prostate cancer. This theory may explain why certain fats—and particularly saturated fats, which are found in animal products—may put men at higher risk of prostate cancer.

The fourth and final hypothesis states that men who consume large amounts of dietary fat suffer more oxidative damage. Oxidative damage is the result of a process of cellular aging. In the natural process of oxidation, free radical molecules are formed. These molecules do damage to cellular structures and important pathways that tend to prevent the development of cancers in general. The prostate is particularly susceptible to oxidative damage—hence the potential benefits of anti-oxidants in preventing prostate cancer, discussed below.

There is some evidence from clinical studies that men with diets low in fat are at lower risk of prostate cancer, particularly the advanced stage of the disease, than those with diets rich in fat.

In one study in Quebec, the time to death due to prostate cancer in men with established prostate cancer was three times shorter in men with diets rich in fat than in those with diets low in fat. Although there is no definitive proof that lowering fat intake can alter the outcome, it can be argued that this evidence supports the recommendation that men with prostate cancer or at high risk for the disease make a reasonable effort to limit dietary fat consumption to about 20 to 25 percent of their total calories.

VITAMIN E

Vitamin E is a major intracellular anti-oxidant. It is typically found in plant-derived oils but is commonly taken in the form of an alphatocopheral dietary supplement. Vitamin E has a long history of safety, although recent studies have questioned the safety of larger doses.

A variety of studies have shown vitamin E to slow the growth of human prostate cancer cells and the rate of cellular turnover. In one large randomized trial, men who were randomly assigned to receive vitamin E demonstrated a one-third lower risk of developing prostate cancer four years after the intervention and a 42 percent lower risk of death from prostate cancer six years after the study began. This study was conducted in Finland on smokers, who seem to derive a particular benefit from vitamin E.

A number of large clinical trials are currently looking at the role of vitamin E in preventing prostate cancer and the conversion of pre-prostate cancer (also known as PIN). These studies are taking place in North America and one is sponsored by the National Cancer Institute of Canada (NCIC). The results of these studies have been largely disappointing. In the NCIC study of men with high-grade prostatic intraepithelial neoplasia (HGPIN), a powder containing vitamin E demonstrated no benefit in terms of lowering the chances that men with the condition will get cancer.

Furthermore, the large-scale SELECT study demonstrated no benefit from 400 IU of vitamin E in terms of preventing prostate cancer. Indeed, a recent reanalysis suggests that there may even be a higher chance of getting prostate cancer if vitamin E is taken. Given this newer evidence it seems prudent to take no more than the recommended daily allowance of vitamin E.

SELENIUM

Selenium is a micronutrient commonly found in the soil in certain parts of the world. Aside from Brazil nuts (which are native to Brazil) there is no consistent source of dietary selenium. Recent studies have looked at the efficacy of selenium in preventing a variety of cancers, including prostate cancer. In one large study conducted in the southwestern United States, the administration of selenium to men coincided with a dramatic 70 percent reduction in prostate cancer development at ten years. This was also a double-blind trial, which adds credence to the results. Additional bodies of scientific knowledge, based on both epidemiology and basic laboratory studies, have shown the positive impact of selenium on DNA repair, slowing cell turnover and inducing cell death. These effects have been noted in prostate cancer cells in particular.

Selenium must be used with caution, however. Large doses can cause selenosis, and recent studies suggest that long-time consumers of selenium may be at higher risk of secondary skin cancers and even diabetes. The current recommendation for patients is 100 to 200 micrograms of selenium per day. As with vitamin E, major clinical trials studying men with HGPIN and prostate cancer prevention in general have been negative, indicating no benefit. Clearly more study is needed. It is difficult to recommend supplemental selenium given the current level of evidence.

LYCOPENE

Lycopene is another key intracellular anti-oxidant. Major sources of lycopene are processed tomato products such as tomato juice, soup, paste and sauce. Other sources of lycopene include watermelon and guava. About 50 milligrams of lycopene per day are recommended.

Several studies have shown that lycopene supplementation can have a beneficial impact on a variety of aspects of prostate cancer, including slowing tumour growth and causing the death of established human prostate cancer cells. A variety of studies of lycopene are currently underway, although none are randomized trials. In a recent study conducted by a group at the University of Toronto, lycopene in combination with selenium and vitamin E was shown to be particularly effective in reducing cell turnover, slowing tumour growth and causing cell death.

Lycopene is available as a supplement. However, consuming one and a half litres of tomato juice per day makes supplements unnecessary. If a supplement is desired, 20 to 50 milligrams per day are suggested.

SOY PROTEIN

Because of the low rates of prostate cancer in China and Japan, where soy is commonly consumed, there has been great interest in studying soy for its cancer-fighting properties. Soy is known to contain natural estrogenic compounds, which may balance the androgens to prevent prostate cancer. There are also some additional non-hormonal mechanisms by which soy may inhibit cancer development and progression. In fact, a large new class of chemotherapy agents work by inhibiting pathways in a way similar to soy. A variety of definitive soy studies are now underway. The current recommendation is 50 to 100 milligrams of soy protein isolate per day for patients who wish to take this type of therapy to complement traditional forms of prostate cancer treatment.

Complications of soy intake can include bloating, intestinal gas and minor weight gain. Further studies will establish the role of soy in prostate cancer in the coming years. To date though, supplemental studies of soy have not demonstrated a benefit in terms of slowing the progression from HGPIN to invasive cancer. Other studies will be forthcoming.

GREEN TEA

As with soy, there is great interest in green tea and its medicinal properties. Green tea is rich in catechins, which are compounds with significant anti-tumour properties. A small study recently conducted in Italy on men with pre-cancer suggests that green tea supplementation may inhibit the progression from pre-cancer to cancer. Although the study is small, it suggests that consuming green tea might be beneficial to men with prostate cancer.

INSULIN RESISTANCE

Obesity and diabetes continue to be a major problem in the Western world, particularly in North America. Rates of obesity are skyrocketing, as are rates of diabetes. Type II diabetes is actually not a condition of insulin deficiency but rather one in which the cells become resistant to the effect of insulin. Recent studies looking at the impact of carbohydrates on prostate cancer progression seem to suggest that tumours grow more slowly in animals with low insulin levels. Thus, low carbohydrate intake seems to slow the growth of tumours. Although further work is needed, the implication is that the intake of complex carbohydrates should be increased and the intake of simple sugars, such as those commonly found in candy, juice and sugared drinks, should be minimized and perhaps avoided altogether if possible. Indeed, the glycemic index is what seems to be driving this process. Insulin has been known to cause cancer cells to grow faster, and it is believed that this is the mechanism at work here. Patients are therefore encouraged to minimize their intake of simple sugars.

FLAX SEED

Flax seed contains a variety of beneficial compounds, including phytoestrogens and fatty acids that may be beneficial in the context of prostate cancer. Additional studies are currently underway. At this point, patients are encouraged to take flax seed, even though the body of scientific literature on this food substance is not nearly as conclusive as that on the other strategies mentioned here.

VITAMIN D

Vitamin D is actually not a vitamin but a hormone. It is synthesized under the influence of sunlight. The majority of Canadians, particularly the elderly, are vitamin D deficient, especially during winter. In light of this, numerous studies have suggested that vitamin D deficiency may be associated with prostate cancer development and/or progression. Vitamin D supplements are recommended for all Canadians, including those with or at a high risk of prostate cancer. Doses of up to 1500 IU appear to be safe and are recommended.

KEY POINTS TO REMEMBER

- Diet plays an important role in the development and/or the progression of prostate cancer. The dietary elements described in this chapter can help patients obtain tangible results, either by preventing prostate cancer or by slowing its progress.

- As mentioned, major clinical trials have largely been disappointing in this field. Despite the negative studies, general healthy eating is strongly advised. This includes low amounts of dietary fat, minimal red meat intake and diets rich in fruits, vegetables and low glycemic foods.

- Dietary manipulation can play a role in preventing cardiovascular disease and other types of cancers (colon cancer, for example). It should also be remembered that many men who are diagnosed with prostate cancer are cured or are at low risk of death from the disease. There may be tangible benefits for such men from dietary changes that help prevent other diseases.

- More research is needed. For now, however, it is recommended that patients make smart choices about their diets.

USEFUL ADDRESSES

CANADA

Canadian Cancer Society (CCS)
National Office
55 St. Clair Avenue West, Suite 300
Toronto, Ontario M4V 2Y7
1-416 961-7223
Toll-free cancer information and support: 1-888-939-3333
(TTY 1-866-786-3934)
Consult the website for contact information for offices across Canada.
www.cancer.ca

A national, community-based organization of volunteers whose mission is the eradication of cancer and the enhancement of the quality of life of people living with cancer. The CCS offers a wide range of information as well as support programs for people living with cancer, including prostate cancer.

Prostate Cancer Canada (PCC)
2 Lombard Street, 3rd Floor
Toronto, Ontario M5C 1M1
1-416-441-2131
Toll-free: 1-888-255-0333
www.prostatecancer.ca

Prostate Cancer Canada is the leading national foundation dedicated to eliminating the most common cancer in men through research, support, education, awareness and advocacy.

The Prostate Cancer Canada Network, a PCC entity, comprises over 70 prostate cancer support groups from coast to coast that provide services at the grassroots level, through monthly peer meetings, special educational events, outreach programs and presentations to service clubs, community health fairs and more.

Prostate Cancer Information Service
Talk to an information specialist today!
1-855-PCC-INFO (1-855-722-4636)
support@prostatecancer.ca

Patients, caregivers, the public and healthcare professionals can contact prostate cancer specialists directly and free of charge.

The Prostate Centre
Princess Margaret Hospital
610 University Avenue, 4th Floor
Toronto, Ontario M5G 2M9
1-416-946-2000 (hospital)
www.prostatecentre.ca

The Prostate Centre provides support and prevention services for men living with prostate cancer and their families. Among other things, men who visit the centre can consult a specialized library and speak to volunteers from the prostate cancer support group Man to Man. The website provides information for the public about prostate cancer.

QUÉBEC

Canadian Cancer Society (CCS)
Regional Office
5151 de l'Assomption Blvd.
Montréal, Québec H1T 4A9
514-255-5151
Toll-free: 1-888-939-3333
The website gives contact information for regional offices across Québec.
www.cancer.ca

A national, community-based organization of volunteers whose mission is the eradication of cancer and the enhancement of the quality of life of people living with cancer. The CCS offers a wide range of information as well as support programs for people living with cancer, including prostate cancer.

Canadian Urological Association (CUA)
185 Dorval Avenue, Suite 401
Dorval, Québec H9S 5J9
514-395-0376
www.cua.org

The physicians who are members of the association are responsible for the information on line at cua.org in the patient information section, where brochures providing reliable information for patients and their families are available.

Fondation québécoise du cancer
2075 de Champlain
Montréal, Québec H2L 2T1
514-527-2194
Toll-free: 1-877-336-4443
Service Info-cancer: 1-800-363-0063
The website provides contact information for regional centres.
www.fqc.qc.ca

The foundation's resources are used to provide support for people living with cancer and their families. Lodging, information and accompaniment are the key services offered.

Groupe de soutien du cancer de la prostate
Notre-Dame Hospital, CHUM
1051 Sanguinet Street, Room D01-3002
Montréal, Québec H2X 3E4
514-890-8000, ext. 24619
www.soutienprostatechum.org

The mission of Le Groupe de soutien du cancer de la prostate is to provide moral support for people with prostate cancer and their significant family or friends. The Groupe provides information and services that help in gaining a better understanding of the disease, its evolution and the different treatments available. Activities and services include a telephone helpline, conferences and workshops.

Fondation Virage pour le soutien au cancer
Centre intégré de cancérologie du CHUM
1051 Sanguinet Street, Room C14-7065
Montréal, Québec H2X 3E4
514-890-8000, ext. 28139
www.viragecancer.org

The foundation's mission is to develop assistance programs and provide services, resources and activities for people with cancer and their significant family or friends, offering accompaniment and support throughout the illness.

PROCURE - The Force Against Prostate Cancer
1320 Graham Blvd., Suite 110
Mount Royal, Québec H3P 3C8
Toll-free 24/7: 1-855-899-2873
info@procure.ca
www.procure.ca

PROCURE's mission is to provide scientists and the community with the means to better prevent and cure prostate cancer.

PROCURE is the only charitable organization in Québec exclusively dedicated to the fight against prostate cancer through research, outreach, education and support for men suffering from prostate cancer and their families. Contact PROCURE to find out about the organization's research biobank, conference series, outreach activities, support groups and telephone support from a health professional or a prostate cancer survivor.

Québec Urological Association (AUQ)
2 Complexe Desjardins, Tour de l'est, 32nd Floor
Montréal, Québec H5B 1G8
514-350-5131
Toll-free: 1-800-561-0703
www.auq.org

Among other things, this association of Québec urologists maintains a website that provides information about prostate cancer for patients and the general public.

GLOSSARY*

Abdomen: the part of the body below the chest that contains organs like the intestines, the liver, the kidneys, the stomach, the bladder, and the prostate.

Ablation: reduction of; e.g., in the management of prostate cancer, hormonal ablation means the use of hormonal techniques to reduce the spread of prostate cancer cells and cryoablation means the use of deep freezing techniques to reduce the number of live prostate and prostate cancer cells.

Active surveillance: active observation and regular monitoring of a patient (DRE, PSA level and re-biopsy) without aggressive treatment until there is evidence of disease progression.

Acute prostatitis: prostate infection characterized by the sudden flare-up of severe symptoms such as high fever and a burning sensation when urinating.

---

* Published with the kind permission of Procure.
  The website www.procure.ca is dedicated to all people seeking information on the prevention, diagnosis, treatment and eventual cure of prostate cancer.

Adenocarcinoma: a form of cancer that develops from a malignant abnormality in the glandular cells lining an organ such as the prostate; almost all prostate cancers are adenocarcinomas.

Adjuvant: added on; e.g., adjuvant hormone therapy is hormone therapy added on to another form of therapy.

Adrenal: the two adrenal glands are located above the kidneys; they produce a variety of different hormones, including sex hormones – e.g., adrenal androgens.

Adrenalectomy: the surgical removal of one or both adrenal glands.

Age-adjusted: modified to take account of the age of an individual or group of individuals; for example, prostate cancer survival data and average normal PSA values can be adjusted according to the ages of groups of men.

Alphablockers: pharmaceutical drugs that act on the prostate by relaxing certain types of muscle tissue; these pharmaceutical drugs are often used in the treatment of BPH.

Analog: a synthetic chemical or pharmaceutical drug that behaves very much like a normal chemical in the body.

Anandron: trade or brand name for nilutamide.

Anatomy: the study of the structure of the body and the relationship between its parts.

Androgen: a hormone which is responsible for male characteristics and the development and function of male sexual organs (e.g. testosterone).

Anemia: a reduction below normal in the oxygen-carrying capacity of the blood.

Anesthesia: the loss of feeling or sensation caused by a drug or gas. General anesthesia causes loss of consciousness with local anesthesia numbs only a certain area.

Aneuploid: having an abnormal number of sets of chromosomes; e.g., tetraploid means having two paired sets of chromosomes, which is twice as many as normal (see also "Diploid").

Anterior: The front; e.g., the anterior of the prostate is the part of the prostate that faces forward.

Anti-androgen: a compound (usually a synthetic pharmaceutical drug) which blocks or otherwise interferes with the normal action of androgens. Usually used in combination with orchiectomy or LHRH analogs.

Antibiotic: a pharmaceutical that can kill certain types of bacteria.

Antibody: protein produced by the immune system as a defense against an invading or "foreign" material or substance (for example, when you get a cold, your body produces antibodies to the cold virus).

Anticholinergic: an agent that blocks nerves that are not under conscious control.

Anti-coagulant: a pharmaceutical drug that helps to stop the blood from clotting.

Antigen: "foreign" material introduced into the body (a virus or bacterium, for example) or other material which the immune system considers to be "foreign" because it is not part of the body's normal biology (e.g., prostate cancer cells).

Anus: the opening of the rectum.

Apex: the tip or bottom of the prostate, i.e., the part of the prostate farthest away from the bladder.

Artificial sphincter: prosthesis or artificial device sometimes used to treat incontinence after prostate surgery.

Aspiration: the use of suction to remove fluid or tissue, usually through a fine needle (e.g., aspiration biopsy).

Asymptomatic: having no recognizable symptoms of a particular disorder.

Base: the base of the prostate is the wide part at the top of the prostate closest to the bladder.

Benign: relatively harmless; not cancerous; not malignant; not potentially fatal.

Benign prostatic hyperplasia: see "BPH".

Bias: a point of view preventing impartial judgment on issues. In clinical trials "blinding" and "randomization" serve to minimize bias.

Bicalutamide: a non-steroidal anti-androgen available in the U.S. and some European countries for the treatment of advanced prostate cancer.

Bilateral: both sides; e.g., a bilateral orchiectomy is an operation in which both testicles are removed and a bilateral adrenalectomy involves removal of both adrenal glands.

Biofeedback: a procedure that uses electrodes to help people gain awareness and control of their pelvic muscles.

Biophosphanate: medication used to increase bone density to avoid fracture and decrease the likelihood of bone pain.

Biopsy: sampling of tissue from a particular part of the body (e.g., the prostate) in order to check for abnormalities such as cancer; in the case of prostate cancer, biopsies are usually carried out under ultrasound guidance using a specially designed device known as a prostate biopsy gun.

Bladder: the hollow sac-like organ in which urine is collected and stored in the body.

Blind: a randomized clinical trial is considered blind when the participants do not know whether they are in the group being given the experimental treatment (experimental group) or the group that is receiving the best available standard treatment (control group).

Bone scan: a sensitive technique which uses radiolabelled agents to identify abnormal or cancerous growths within or attached to bone; in the case of prostate cancer, a bone scan is used to identify bony metastases which are definitive for cancer which has escaped from the prostate.

Bowel preparation: the cleaning of the bowels or intestines which is normal prior to abdominal surgery such as radical prostatectomy.

BPH: benign prostatic hyperplasia or enlargement of the prostate occurs in most men age they age; it can cause difficulties for many men (such as the frequent need to urinate at night), which can become severe for some individuals.

Brachytherapy: the implantation of radioactive seeds or pellets which emit low energy radiation in order to kill surrounding tissue (e.g., the prostate, including prostate cancer cells).

Bulbous urethra: enlarged section of the urethra downstream from where the urethra passes through the prostate. Seminal fluid collects in the bulbous urethra before ejaculation.

Buserelin acetate: a luteinizing hormone releasing hormone analog used in the palliative hormonal treatment of advanced prostate cancer and sometimes in the adjuvant and neoadjuvant hormonal treatment of earlier stages of prostate cancer.

C

CAB: complete androgen blockade (see "Maximal androgen deprivation").

Cancer: the growth of abnormal cells in the body in an uncontrolled manner.

Capsule: the fibrous tissue which acts as an outer lining of the prostate.

Carcinoma: another word meaning cancer.

Casodex: brand name or trade name of bicalutamide.

Castration: the use of surgical or medical techniques to lower the level of testosterone in the male to zero or near zero.

Catheter: a hollow (usually plastic) tube that can be used to drain fluids from or inject fluids into the body; in the case of prostate cancer, it is common for patients to have a transurethral catheter to drain urine for some time after treatment by surgery or some forms of radiation therapy.

Chemoprevention: the use of a pharmaceutical drug or other substance to prevent the development of cancer.

Chemotherapy: the use of pharmaceutical drugs to kill cancer cells; in many cases chemotherapeutic agents kill not only cancer cells but also other cells in the body, which makes such agents potentially very dangerous.

Chromosome: threadlike structure in every cell that consists of genes composed of DNA. One human cell normally consists of 46 chromosomes.

CHT: combined hormone therapy or treatment (see "Maximal androgen deprivation").

Clinical trial: a carefully planned experiment to evaluate a treatment or a medication (often a pharmaceutical drug) for an unproven use.

Collagen: colloidal chemical substance made of proteins, sometimes injected into the urinary sphincter region to treat incontinence.

Complication: an unexpected or unwanted effect of a treatment, pharmaceutical drug, or other procedure.

Conformational therapy: the use of careful planning and delivery techniques designed to focus radiation on the areas of the prostate and surrounding tissue that need treatment and protect areas that do not need treatment: three-dimensional conformational therapy is a more sophisticated form of this method.

Congestion: situation characterized by buildup of fluid in some area of the body. In prostate congestion, there is an unrelieved, often painful buildup of prostatic fluid in the prostate, sometimes accounting for cases of prostatosis.

Continence: ability to retain urine.

Contracture: scarring that can occur at the bladder neck after a radical prostatectomy and that results in narrowing of the passage between the bladder and the urethra.

Control group: the group in the clinical trial that receives the best available standard treatment.

Cooperative groups: networks of organizations and researchers at academic and community practices that collaborate to conduct research. Many such cooperative groups exist in Quebec.

Corpus cavernosum: two chambers running the length of a man's penis that fill with blood when he is sexually excited, giving the organ the stiffness required for intercourse.

Corpus spongiosum: a spongy chamber in a man's penis that contains the urethra and fills with blood when he is sexually excited, giving the organ the stiffness required for intercourse.

Cryoablation: see "Cryosurgery".

Cryosurgery: the use of liquid nitrogen to freeze a particular organ to extremely low temperatures to kill the tissue, including any cancerous tissue.

Cryotherapy: see "Cryosurgery".

CT scan: computerized tomography (also known as computerized axial tomography or CAT scan), a method of combining images from multiple X-rays under the control of a computer to produce sophisticated cross-sectional or three-dimensional pictures of the internal organs, which can be used to identify abnormalities.

Cystoscope: an instrument used by physicians to look inside the bladder and the urethra.

Cystoscopy: the use of a cystoscope to look inside the bladder and the urethra.

Debulking: reduction of the volume of cancer by one of several techniques; most frequently used to imply surgical debulking.

DES: see "Diethylstilbestrol."

DHT: see "Dihydrotestosterone."

Diagnosis: the evaluation of signs, symptoms, and selected test results by a physician to determine the physical and biological causes of the signs and symptoms and whether a specific disease or disorder is involved.

Diethylstilbestrol: a female hormone commonly used in the 1960's and 1970's for treatment of prostate cancer.

Differentiation: the process of changing from an original unspecialized form to a different, more specialized form; e.g. the differences between prostate cancer cells are examined under the microscope as a method to grade the severity of the disease.

Digital rectal examination: the use by a physician of a lubricated and gloved finger inserted into the rectum to feel for abnormalities of the prostate and rectum.

Dihydrotestosterone: the male hormone active in the prostate; it is produced when an enzyme in the prostate transforms testosterone.

Diploid: having one complete set of normally paired chromosomes, i.e., a normal amount of DNA.

DNA: deoxyribonucleic acid; the basic biologically active molecule that defines the physical development and growth of nearly all living organisms.

Double-blinded study: a form of clinical trial in which neither the medical staff nor the participants know the actual treatment which any individual participant is receiving; double-blind trials are a way of minimizing the effects of the personal opinions of patients and physicians on the results of the trial.

Doubling time: the time that it takes a particular focus of cancer to double in size.

Downsizing: the use of hormonal or other forms of management to reduce the volume of prostate cancer in and /or around the prostate prior to attempted curative treatment.

Downstaging: the use of hormonal or other forms of management in the attempt to lower the clinical stage of prostate cancer prior to attempted curative treatment (e.g., from stage T3a to stage T2b); this technique is highly controversial.

DRE: see "Digital rectal examination".

Drip collector: collecting device, either internal or external, to collect urine from an incontinent person.

Dysplasia: see "Prostatic intraepithelial neoplasia".

Ejaculate: the sperm-containing fluid (semen) that is emitted during ejaculation. Ejaculate generally contains sperm originating in the testicles and seminal fluid originating in the testicles, seminal vesicles, and prostate.

Ejaculation: sudden discharge of semen during sexual intercourse or masturbation.

Eligard: brand or trade name of leuprolide acetate in the U.S. and Canada.

Emcyt: brand or trade name of estramustine phosphate in the U.S.

Enzyme: a protein produced in cells, that speeds up the rate of biological reactions without itself being used up.

Epididymis: two common-shaped tubes inside the scrotum that surround each testicle.

Erectile dysfunction: the inability to obtain or maintain an erection sufficient for penetration. This condition must be persistent for a period of at least three months before being considered a dysfunction.

Erection: a mechanism that allows for rigidity, such as the result of an increased blood flow to the penis.

Estramustine phosphate: a chemotherapeutic agent used in the treatment of some patients with late stage prostate cancer.

Estrogen: one of the most important female hormones; certain estrogens (e.g. diethylstilbestrol) are used by some physicians in treatment of prostate cancer.

Eulexin: the brand or trade name of flutamide in the U.S.

Experimental: an unproven (or even untested) technique or procedure; note that certain experimental treatments are commonly used in the management of prostate cancer.

External beam: a form of radiation therapy in which the radiation is delivered by a machine pointed at the area to be radiated.

Fibrosis: the formation of a scar.

Fistula: an abnormal passage or communication, usually between two internal organs or leading from an internal organ to the surface of the body.

5-alph reductase: an enzyme found in the prostate that controls conversion of testosterone into dihydrotestosterone (DHT). When the action of this enzyme is blocked, production of DHT is inhibited, stopping growth of a benign prostate tumour.

Flutamide: an anti-androgen used in the palliative hormonal treatment of advanced prostate cancer and sometimes in the adjuvant and neoadjuvant hormonal treatment of earlier stages of prostate cancer.

Foley catheter: type of catheter named for its inventor, with a balloon at the end inserted into the body. The balloon holds the catheter in place. A Foley is usually inserted through the penis to drain urine after prostate surgery.

Free PSA: PSA that is not bound to proteins.

Frequency: the need to urinate often.

Gastrointestinal: related to the digestive system and/or the intestines.

Gene: one of many discrete units of hereditary information located on the chromosomes and consisting of DNA.

Gene therapy: a new type of treatment in which defective genes are replaced with normal ones.

Genital system: the biological system which, in males, includes the testicles, the vas deferens, the seminal vesicles, the prostate, and the penis.

Genito-urinary system: the combined genital and urinary systems, also known as the genito-urinary tract.

Gland: a structure or organ that produces a substance used in another part of the body.

Glaucoma: a group of eye diseases characterized by an increase in intraocular pressure, causing defects in the field of vision.

Gleason: name of physician who developed the Gleason grading system commonly used to grade prostate cancer.

Goserelin acetate: a luteinizing hormone releasing hormone analog used in the palliative hormonal treatment of advanced prostate cancer and sometimes in the adjuvant and neoadjuvant hormonal treatment of earlier stages of prostate cancer.

Grade: a means of describing the potential degree of severity of a cancer based on the appearance of cancer cells under a microscope; see also "Gleason".

Gynecomastia: enlargement or tenderness of the male breasts or nipples.

Hematospermia: the occurrence of blood in the semen.

Hematuria: the occurrence of blood in the urine.

Heredity: the historical distribution of biological characteristics through a group of related individuals via their DNA.

Hereditary: inherited from one's parents and earlier generations.

Histology: the study of the appearance and behaviour of tissue, usually carried out under a microscope by a pathologist (who is a physician) or a histologist (who is not necessarily a physician).

Homogeneous: uniform, of the same kind.

Hormone: a biologically active chemical responsible for the development of secondary sexual characteristics.

Hormone therapy: the use of hormones, hormone analogs, and certain surgical techniques to treat disease (in this case advanced prostate cancer) either on their own or in combination with other hormones or in combination with other methods of treatment.

Hot flash: the sudden sensation of warmth in the face, neck and upper body, a side effect of many forms of hormone therapy.

Hyperplasia: enlargement of an organ or tissue because of an increase in the number of cells in that organ or tissue; see also "BPH."

Imaging: a technique or method allowing a physician to see something that would not normally be visible.

Immune system: the biological system that protects a person or animal from the effects of foreign materials such as bacteria viruses, cancer cells, and other things that might make that person or animal sick.

Implant: a device inserted into the body in order to replace or substitute for an ability that has been lost; for example, a penile implant is a device that can be surgically inserted into the penis to provide rigidity for intercourse.

Impotence: the inability to have or to maintain an erection.

Incidental: insignificant or irrelevant; for example, incidental prostate cancer (also known as latent prostate cancer) is a form of prostate cancer that is of no clinical significance to the patient in whom it is discovered.

Incontinence: leaking of or inability to control any substance, but commonly the leaking of or inability to control urine (properly called urinary incontinence).

Indication: a reason for doing something or taking some action; also used to mean the approved clinical application of a pharmaceutical drug.

Infertility: in a man with prostate problems, the inability to father a child due to prostate infection or retrograde ejaculation.

Inflammation: any form of swelling or pain or irritation.

Informed consent: in the case of a clinical trial, it means that you know what the trial is about, you understand why it is being conducted and why you have been invited to take part, and you appreciate exactly how you will be involved.

Interstitial: within a particular organ; for example, interstitial prostate radiation therapy is radiation therapy applied within the prostate using implanted radioactive pellets or seeds (see also "Brachytherapy").

Interstitial cystitis: a chronic inflammatory condition of the bladder.

Intravenous: into a vein.

Intravenous pyelogram: a procedure that introduces a radioactive substance into the urinary tract in order to allow the physician a superior image of the tract by taking an X-ray.

Invasive: requiring an incision or the insertion of an instrument or substance into the body.

IVP: see "Intravenous pyelogram".

Kegel exercises: a set of exercises designed to improve the strength of the muscles of the pelvic floor, in order to augment urinary control and prevent leakage.

Kidney: one of a pair of organs whose primary function is to filter the fluids passing through the body.

Laparoscopic lymph node dissection: test procedure using a device called a laparoscope that involves the removal of tissue through small incisions for later examination of possibly cancerous lymph nodes in the vicinity of the prostate.

Laparoscopy: a technique allowing the physician to observe internal organs directly through a piece of optical equipment inserted directly into the body through a small surgical incision.

Latent: insignificant or irrelevant; for example, latent prostate cancer (also known as incidental prostate cancer) is a form of prostate cancer of no clinical significance to the patient in whom it is discovered.

Leuprolide acetate: a luteinizing hormone-releasing hormone analog used in the palliative hormonal treatment of advanced prostate cancer and sometimes in the adjuvant and neoadjuvant hormonal treatment of earlier stages of prostate cancer.

LH-RH: see "Luteinizing hormone releasing hormone".

LH-RH analog: a man-made hormone that is chemically similar to LH-RH.

Libido: interest in sexual activity.

Lobe: one of the two sides of an organ that clearly has two sides (e.g. the prostate or the brain).

Localized: restricted to a well-defined area.

Lupron: brand or trade name of leuprolide acetate in the U.S. and Canada.

Luteinizing hormone-releasing hormone: a hormone responsible for stimulating the production of testosterone in the body.

Lycopene: the major red pigment in some fruit.

Lymph: the clear fluid in which all of the cells in the body are constantly bathed, also known as the lymphatic fluid.

Lymphadenectomy: a surgical procedure in which the lymph nodes are dissected.

Lymph node: any of the many small structures that filter lymph and produce lymphocytes. Lymph nodes are concentrated in several areas of the body, such as the armpit, groin, and neck.

Lymphocyte: a white blood cell that normally makes up 25 percent of the total white blood cell count but increases in the presence of infection. Lymphocytes aid in the protection of the body against illness.

MAB: maximal androgen blockade (see "Maximal androgen deprivation").

MAD: see "Maximal androgen deprivation."

Magnetic resonance imaging: a technique allowing sophisticated vertical, cross-sectional, and even three-dimensional images of organs inside the body based on the electromagnetic properties of different atomic particles as opposed to X-rays.

Male sling: surgery whereby a sling is used to compress the urethra to stop any leakage of urine during such activities as coughing, sneezing or exercising.

Malignancy: a growth or tumour composed of cancerous cells.

Malignant: cancerous.

Margin: normally used to mean the "surgical margin," which is the outer edge of the tissue removed during surgery; if the surgical margin shows no sign of cancer ("negative margins"), then the prognosis is good.

Maximal androgen deprivation: the combined use of two forms of hormonal treatment to block the effects of testosterone and other androgens produced by the adrenal glands (also known by many other names and abbreviations).

Medical oncologist: a doctor who specializes in chemotherapy, which involves the use of drugs to treat cancer. He or she also has a wide experience in relieving physical symptoms such as pain and emotional, psychological or spiritual concerns.

Metastasis: a secondary tumour formed as a result of a cancer cell or cells from the primary tumour site (e.g. the prostate) travelling through the body to a new site and then growing there.

Metastatic: having the characteristics of a secondary tumour.

Metastron: the brand or trade name of strontium-89 in the U.S.

Misstaging: the assignment of an incorrect clinical stage at initial diagnosis because of the difficulty of assessing the available information with accuracy.

Mixed incontinence: exhibiting symptoms of both stress and urge incontinence.

Monoclonal: formed from a single group of identical cells.

MRI: see "Magnetic resonance imaging."

Multi-centre clinical trial: also called multi-site clinical trial; trial that takes place at many different sites at the same time.

Myasthenia gravis: disease whose characteristic feature is easy fatigue of certain voluntary muscle groups on repeated use.

Negative: the term used to describe a test result that does not show the presence of the substance or material for which the test was carried out; for example, a negative bone scan would show no sign of bone metastases.

Neoadjuvant: added before; for example, neoadjuvant hormone therapy is therapy given prior to another form of treatment such as a radical prostatectomy.

Neoplasia: the growth of cells under conditions that would tend to prevent the development of normal tissue (e.g. a cancer).

Neoplasm: any abnormal growth in the body. May be benign or malignant.

Nerve sparing: term used to describe a type of prostatectomy in which the surgeon saves the nerves that affect sexual and related functions.

Neurogenic bladder: a dysfunction due to a malfunction of the nerves responsible for the control of bladder function.

Nilutamide: an anti-androgen, still experimental in the U.S., but available in Canada and some other countries.

Nitrates: medications used to treat chest pain.

Nocturia: the need to urinate frequently at night.

Non-invasive: not requiring any incision nor the insertion of an instrument or substance into the body.

Oncologist: a physician who specializes in the treatment of various types of cancer.

Orchiectomy: the surgical removal of the testicles.

Organ: a group of tissues that work in concert to carry out a specific set of functions (e.g. the heart or the lungs or the prostate).

Osteoporosis: reduction of bone mass leading to fractures after minimal trauma.

Overactive bladder: a condition characterized by involuntary bladder muscle contractions that cannot be suppressed.

Overflow incontinence: the loss of small amounts of urine from a bladder that is always full. Also called paradoxical incontinence.

Overstaging: the assignment of an overly high clinical stage at initial diagnosis because of the difficulty of assessing the available information with accuracy (e.g. stage T3b as opposed to stage T2b).

Palliative: designed to relieve a particular problem or problems without necessarily solving them; for example, palliative therapy is given in order to relieve symptoms and improve quality of life but not to cure the patient.

Palpable: capable of being felt during a physical examination by an experienced physician; in the case of prostate cancer, this normally refers to some form of abnormality of the prostate that can be felt during a digital rectal examination.

PAP: see "Prostatic acid phosphatase."

Pathologist: a physician who specializes in the examination of tissues and blood samples to help decide what diseases are present and how they should be treated.

Pelvic floor muscles exercises: see "Kegel exercises."

Pelvic node dissection: removal of the lymph nodes in the pelvis.

Pelvis: that part of the skeleton that joins the lower limbs of the body.

Penile: of the penis.

Penile implant: prosthesis or artificial device used to treat impotence. When surgically inserted into the penis, it provides sufficient rigidity for vaginal penetration and sustained sexual intercourse.

Penis: the male organ used in urination and intercourse.

Perineal: of the perineum.

Perineal prostatectomy: surgical removal of the prostate through an incision between the scrotum and anus.

Perineum: the area of the body between the scrotum and the rectum.

Peripheral: outside the central region.

Peyronie's disease: a disease of unknown cause in which plaques form around the corpus cavernosum of the penis, causing deviation and painful erection.

PIN: see "Prostatic intraepithelial neoplasia."

Pituitary gland: gland at the base of the brain that produces hormones stimulating release of other hormones, including testosterone.

Placebo: a safe but inactive (fake) pill, liquid or powder that is used as a basis for comparison with pharmaceuticals in research studies.

Ploidy: a term used to describe the number of sets of chromosomes in a cell; see also "Diploid and aneuploid."

Positive: the term used to describe a test result that shows the presence of the substance or material for which the test was carried out; for example, a positive bone scan would show signs of bone metastases.

Posterior: the rear; for example, the posterior of the prostate is the part of the prostate that faces a man's back.

Priapism: a persistent abnormal erection of the penis accompanied by pain and tenderness that requires medical attention.

Prognosis: the patient's potential clinical outlook based on the status and probable course of his disease.

Progression: continuing growth or regrowth of the cancer.

Prostascint scan: a scan that uses low-level radioactive material to find cancer that has spread beyond the prostate.

Prostate: the spherical gland, about the size of a walnut, surrounding the urethra and immediately below the bladder in males. Secretes part of the seminal fluid and controls urinary flow.

Prostate specific antigen (PSA): a protein made by the prostate gland and detected in the blood. Its presence increases in response to the presence of foreign materials such as prostate cancer cells; it is used to detect potential problems in the prostate gland.

Prostate specific antigen density (PSAD): metric determined by dividing the PSA number by the prostate volume (its size as measured by transrectal ultrasound).

Prostatectomy: a surgical removal of the prostate gland; see also "Radical prostatectomy."

Prostatic acid phosphatase (PAP): an enzyme test now used only rarely to decide whether prostate cancer has escaped from the prostate.

Prostatic intraepithelial neoplasia: also called prostatic intraductal neoplasia. a pathologically identifiable condition believed to be a possible precursor of prostate cancer; also known more simply as dysplasia by many physicians.

Prostatitis: infection or inflammation of the prostate gland.

Prostatosis: chronic pain of the prostate.

Prosthesis: a man-made device used to replace a normal body part or function.

Protocol: a precise set of methods by which a research study is to be carried out.

PSA: see "Prostate specific antigen."

PSAD: see "Prostate specific antigen density."

Quality of life: an evaluation of health status relative to the patient's age, expectations, and physical and mental capabilities.

R

Radiation oncologist: a physician who has received special training regarding the treatment of cancers with different types of radiation.

Radiation therapy: (also known as radiotherapy) the use of X-rays in an attempt to destroy malignant tissues.

Radical prostatectomy: the surgical removal of the prostate and surrounding tissue and structures with the intent to cure the problem believed to be caused by or within the prostate.

Radioisotope: a type of atom (or a chemical made with a type of atom) that emits radioactivity.

Radiologist: physician who specializes in radiology, administering and interpreting X-ray, ultrasound and other imaging studies.

Radiology: a branch of medicine concerned with X-rays, ultrasound and other imaging techniques.

Randomization: the process of assigning patients by a method of chance to different forms of treatment (either the experimental group or the control group) in a research study. A way to prevent bias in research.

Rectum: the final part of the intestines ending at the anus.

Recurrence: the reappearance of disease.

Refractory: resistant to therapy.

Regression: reduction in the size of a single tumour or reduction in the number or size of several tumours.

Remission: the real or apparent disappearance of some or all of the signs and symptoms of cancer.

Resection: surgical removal of tissue.

Resectoscope: instrument inserted through the urethra and used by a urologist to cut out tissue (usually from the prostate) while seeing precisely where he is cutting.

Resistance: (in a medical sense) a patient's ability to fight off a disease as a result of the effectiveness of his (or her) immune system.

Retention: difficulty in initiation of urination or the ability to completely empty the bladder.

Retropubic: behind or posterior to the pubic arch.

Retropubic prostatectomy: prostatectomy in which a surgical incision is made through the abdomen at a point above where the penis enters the body, cutting through the bladder to reach the prostate.

Reverse transcriptase polymerase chain reaction (RTPCR): a technique that allows a physician to search for tiny quantities of a protein, such as PSA, in the blood or other body fluids and tissues.

Risk: the chance or probability that a particular event will or will not happen.

RTPCR: see "Reverse transcriptase polymerase chain reaction."

Salvage: a procedure intended to "rescue" a patient following the failure of a prior treatment, for example a salvage prostatectomy would be the surgical removal of the prostate after the failure of prior radiation therapy or cryosurgery.

Screening: the search for disease, such as cancer, in people without symptoms.

Scrotum: the pouch of skin containing a man's testicles.

Secondary tumour: a tumour that spreads (metastasis) from the site where it started.

Seeds: radioactive pellets implanted in the prostate to destroy cancerous growth.

Selenium: a relatively rare non-metallic element that is found in small quantities in food and that may have some effect in prevention of cancer.

Semen: the whitish, opaque fluid emitted by a male at ejaculation.

Seminal: related to the semen.

Seminal vesicles: glands at the base of the bladder and connected to the prostate that add nutrients to the semen.

Serum: the clear liquid portion of the blood (excluding the blood cells).

Sextant: having six parts; thus, a sextant biopsy is a biopsy requiring six samples.

Side effect: a reaction to a medication or treatment (most commonly used to mean an unnecessary or undesirable effect).

Sign: physical changes that can be observed as a consequence of an illness or disease.

Single-centre clinical trial: also called single-site clinical trial; a trial that takes place at only one site and is initiated by one researcher.

Social worker: an individual who specializes in drawing on community resources to benefit people facing a major life crisis. He or she will help you make adjustments and adapt to changing social and economic environments.

Sphincter: the ring of muscles located around the urethra that regulates the passage of urine.

Stage: a term used to define the size and physical extent of a cancer.

Staging: the process of assigning a stage to a particular cancer in a specific patient in light of all the available information.

Stent: a tube used by a surgeon to drain fluids.

Stress incontinence: leakage of urine as a result of physical exertion such as coughing, sneezing, lifting an object and/or exercising.

Stricture: scarring as a result of a procedure or an injury that constricts the flow of a fluid; for example, a urethral stricture would restrict the flow of urine through the urethra.

Strontium-89: an injectable radioactive product used to relieve bone pain in some patients with prostate cancer that no longer responds to hormones or appropriate forms of chemotherapy.

Subcapsular: under the capsule; for example, a subcapsular orchiectomy is a form of castration in which the contents of each testicle is removed but the testicular capsules are then closed and remain in the scrotum.

Suprapubic: above the pubic arch.

Suprapubic prostatectomy: prostatectomy in which a surgical incision is made through the abdomen at a point above where the penis enters the body, bypassing the bladder as the cut is extended to the prostate.

Suprefact: brand or trade name of buserelin acetate in the U.S. and Canada.

Suture: surgical stitching used in the closure of a cut or incision.

Symptom: a feeling, sensation, or experience associated with or resulting from a physical or mental disorder and noticeable by the patient.

Systemic: throughout the whole body.

TAB: total androgen blockade; see "Maximal androgen deprivation."

Testis: one of two male reproductive glands located inside the scrotum which are the primary source of the male hormone testosterone; plural testes.

Testicle: see "Testis."

Testosterone: the male hormone or androgen that makes up about 90 percent of the androgens in a man's body; it is needed to complete male sexual function and fertility.

Total androgen blockade (TAB): see "Maximal androgen deprivation."

Transition: change; for example, the transition zone of the prostate is the area of the prostate closest to the urethra and has features which distinguish it from the much larger peripheral zone.

Transperineal: through the perineum.

Transrectal: through the rectum.

Transrectal ultrasound: a method of imaging the prostate by inserting an ultrasound probe into the rectum; commonly used to visualize prostate biopsy procedures.

Transurethral: through the urethra.

Transurethral hyperthermia (TH): new treatment for benign prostate enlargement; heat generated by a microwave transmitter alleviates urinary obstruction.

Transurethral incision of the prostate (TUIP): new treatment for benign prostate enlargement; a series of small cuts is made inside the urethra to alleviate urinary obstruction.

Transurethral resection of the prostate (TURP): a surgical procedure in which part of the prostate gland surrounding the urethra is removed using a resectoscope.

Transurethral ultrasound-guided laser prostatectomy: new prostatectomy technique used with benign prostate enlargement; a laser beam guided by an ultrasound image removes excess prostate tissue that interferes with normal urination.

TRUS: see "Transrectal ultrasound."

TUIP: see "Transurethral incision of the prostate."

Tumour: an abnormal tissue growth that can be either benign or malignant.

TURP: see "Transurethral resection of the prostate."

Ultrasound: use of ultra high-frequency sound waves to image internal organs and structures (e.g. a baby in the womb).

Understaging: the assignment of an overly low clinical stage at initial diagnosis because of the difficulty of assessing the available information with accuracy (e.g. stage T2b as opposed to stage T3b).

Unit: a surgical term for a pint (usually of blood).

Ureter: an anatomical tube that drains urine from one of the two kidneys to the bladder.

Urethra: the tube that drains urine from the bladder through the prostate and out through the penis.

Urge incontinence: the leakage of urine that occurs when the bladder has involuntary contractions. There is a strong feeling of having to urinate right away and not making it on time to the toilet.

Urgency: the need to urinate right away.

Urinary system: the group of organs and their interconnections that permit excess, filtered fluids to exit the body; including (in the male) the kidneys, the ureters, the bladder, the urethra and the penis.

Urinary tract infection (UTI): an infection identifiable by the presence of bacteria in the urine; may be associated with fever, or a burning pain on urination.

Urologist: a doctor trained first as a surgeon who specializes in disorders of the genito-urinary system.

UTI: see "Urinary tract infection."

Vas deferens: tube through which sperm travel from the testes to the prostate prior to ejaculation.

Vasectomy: operation to make a man sterile by cutting the vas deferens, thus preventing passage of sperm from the testes to the prostate.

Vesicle: a small saclike part (e.g. seminal vesicle) containing fluid.

Watchful waiting: follow-up of patients with prostate cancer until symptoms appear or the cancer spreads, at which time hormone therapy is usually given to reduce symptoms and disease progression.

X-ray: a type of radiation used to make images of the internal structures of the body and in treatment of malignant diseases.

Zoladex: brand or trade name of goserelin acetate in the U.S. and Canada.

Zone: part or area of an organ.

Set in Univers Light
11/14 and printed by
Imprimerie HLN
Sherbrooke, Québec
in January 2019 for
Annika Parance Publishing.